Chest Imaging Cases

Published and Forthcoming books in the
Cases in Radiology **series:**

Chest Imaging Cases

Sanjeev Bhalla, MD

Associate Professor, Radiology
Chief, Cardiothoracic Imaging Section
Mallinckrodt Institute of Radiology
Washington University School of Medicine in St. Louis
St. Louis, Missouri

Cylen Javidan-Nejad, MD

Assistant Professor, Radiology
Mallinckrodt Institute of Radiology
Washington University School of Medicine in St. Louis
St. Louis, Missouri

Kristopher W. Cummings, MD

Assistant Professor, Radiology
Mallinckrodt Institute of Radiology
Washington University School of Medicine in St. Louis
St. Louis, Missouri

Andrew J. Bierhals, MD

Assistant Professor, Radiology
Mallinckrodt Institute of Radiology
Washington University School of Medicine in St. Louis
St. Louis, Missouri

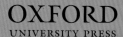

OXFORD
UNIVERSITY PRESS

OXFORD
UNIVERSITY PRESS

Oxford University Press, Inc., publishes works that further
Oxford University's objective of excellence
in research, scholarship, and education.

Oxford   New York
Auckland   Cape Town   Dar es Salaam   Hong Kong   Karachi
Kuala Lumpur   Madrid   Melbourne   Mexico City   Nairobi
New Delhi   Shanghai   Taipei   Toronto

With offices in
Argentina   Austria   Brazil   Chile   Czech Republic   France   Greece
Guatemala   Hungary   Italy   Japan   Poland   Portugal   Singapore
South Korea   Switzerland   Thailand   Turkey   Ukraine   Vietnam

Published by Oxford University Press, Inc.
198 Madison Avenue, New York, New York 10016
www.oup.com

Oxford is a registered trademark of Oxford University Press

Library of Congress Cataloging-in-Publication Data

Chest imaging cases / Sanjeev Bhalla . . . [et al.].
   p. ; cm. — (Cases in radiology)
 Includes bibliographical references and index.
 ISBN 978-0-19-539453-5 (pbk. : alk. paper)
1. Chest—Radiography—Case studies. 2. Diagnosis, Differential—Case studies.
I. Bhalla, Sanjeev. II. Title. III. Series: Cases in radiology.
 [DNLM: 1. Diagnostic Imaging—Case Reports.
2. Thoracic Diseases—diagnosis—Case Reports. WF 975]
 RC941.C47 2012
 617.5'40757—dc22

                                               2011012552

This material is not intended to be, and should not be considered, a substitute for medical or other professional advice. Treatment for the conditions described in this material is highly dependent on the individual circumstances. And, while this material is designed to offer accurate information with respect to the subject matter covered and to be current as of the time it was written, research and knowledge about medical and health issues is constantly evolving and dose schedules for medications are being revised continually, with new side effects recognized and accounted for regularly. Readers must therefore always check the product information and clinical procedures with the most up-to-date published product information and data sheets provided by the manufacturers and the most recent codes of conduct and safety regulation. The publisher and the authors make no representations or warranties to readers, express or implied, as to the accuracy or completeness of this material. Without limiting the foregoing, the publisher and the authors make no representations or warranties as to the accuracy or efficacy of the drug dosages mentioned in the material. The authors and the publisher do not accept, and expressly disclaim, any responsibility for any liability, loss or risk that may be claimed or incurred as a consequence of the use and/or application of any of the contents of this material.

9 8 7 6 5 4 3 2 1
Printed in China
on acid-free paper

To my parents, husband, children, teachers, and colleagues
for their guidance, support, and understanding.
-Cylen Javidan-Nejad

For my children, Elizabeth and Sebastian.
-Andrew J. Bierhals

To my parents for their love and support.
-Kristopher W. Cummings

To my parents, Brahm and Rama, who continue to remind me that
knowledge is only strengthened by being shared.
-Sanjeev Bhalla

Preface and Acknowledgments

We hope that the following cases will serve as a useful foundation for the Radiologist interested in Thoracic Radiology. The following represents the core of what we feel is essential to our field. We attempted to offer practical differential diagnoses and approaches to daily practice that could be used immediately.

We would like to acknowledge our colleagues from the Cardiothoracic Section at the Mallinckrodt Institute of Radiology: Stuart Sagel, Harvey Glazer, Fernando Gutierrez, Janice Semenkovich, Costa Raptis, Dave Gierada, Pam Woodard, Claire Anderson, and Marilyn Siegel. They have been great mentors and teachers who have taught us both in and out of the reading room. They have built a section where the free sharing of cases and knowledge has created a rich environment for the learning of Cardiothoracic Radiology. We are indebted to them for the ability to write a book such as this one. We would also like to thank the many Radiology fellows and residents who continually challenge us in the ability to make findings and understand them. Many of the teaching points in this book come directly from face-to-face readouts.

The Publisher thanks the following for their time and advice:

Mark Anderson, University of Virginia
Sanjeev Bhalla, Mallinckrodt Institute of Radiology, Washington University
Michael Bruno, Penn State Hershey Medical Center
Melissa Rosado de Christenson, St. Luke's Hospital of Kansas City
Rihan Khan, University of Arizona
Angela Levy, Georgetown University
Alexander Mamourian, University of Pennsylvania
Stacy Smith, Brigham and Women's Hospital

Contents

Part 1

Cases that should be Diagnosed on a Chest Radiograph

History

▶ 27-year-old woman with chest tightness and shortness of breath presents to the Emergency Department.

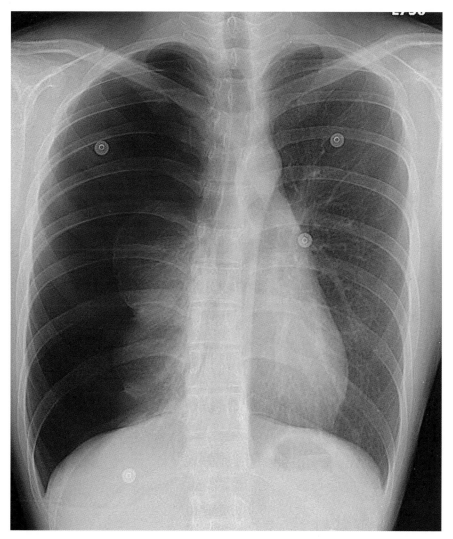

Figure 1.1

Case 1   Tension Pneumothorax

Figure 1.2

Figure 1.3

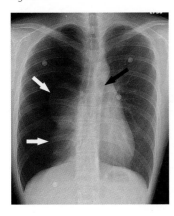

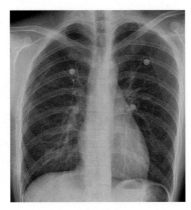

Findings

▶ Initial chest radiograph (Fig. 1.1) clearly demonstrates increased lucency in the right hemothorax with minimal displacement of the right hemidiaphragm inferiorly and shift of the mediastinum leftward. Note the increased distances between the ribs on the right, compared with those on the left. The right lung is partially collapsed.

▶ Visceral pleural surface (white arrows in Fig. 1.2) can be seen as a thin white line, allowing distinction from a skin fold. No pulmonary vessels are seen lateral to the pleural line. The anterior junction line (black arrow in Fig. 1.2) is also displaced leftward.

▶ Once the chest tube is placed, the heart and mediastinum return to their normal location (Fig. 1.3). Note the change in appearance of the right heart border and right hemidiaphragm.

Differential Diagnosis

▶ Tension pneumothorax. There should be no differential diagnosis.

Teaching Points

▶ A tension pneumothorax results in shift of the mediastinum to the contralateral side and the diaphragm inferiorly.

▶ In patients on positive ventilation, the diaphragm may be more displaced than the mediastinum, as the positive ventilation bolsters the unaffected side.

Management

▶ Needs emergent drainage. The mass effect can impede oxygen exchange on the contralateral side and impair venous return to the heart. Left untreated, a tension pneumothorax can result in cardiorespiratory collapse.

▶ When encountered in the reading room, the tension pneumothorax should prompt a phone call to the referring clinician. This phone call should be documented in the radiology report.

Further Reading

Barton ED. Tension pneumothorax. *Curr Opin Pulm Med*. 1999 Jul;5(4):269-274.

Leigh-Smith S, Harris T. Tension pneumothorax—time for a re-think? *Emerg Med J*. 2005 Jan;22(1):8-16.

History

► 19-year-old man after a motor vehicle collision is imaged in the trauma suite.

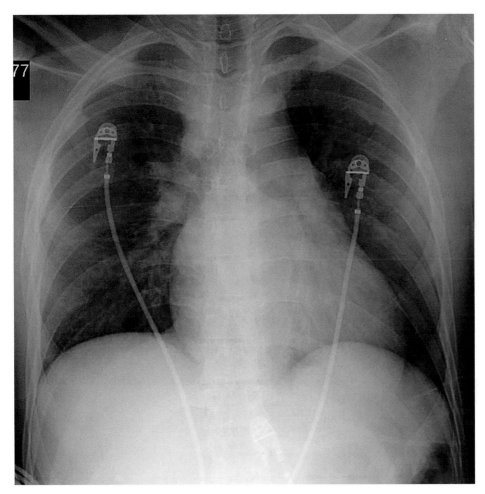

Figure 2.1

Case 2 Pneumothorax with Deep Sulcus Sign

Figure 2.2

Figure 2.3

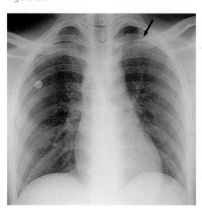 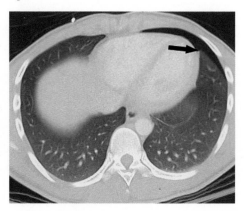

Findings

► Supine radiograph (Fig. 2.1) shows increased lucency at the left base, but no pleural line is seen. The left costophrenic sulcus extends more inferiorly than the right. Wires represent ECG leads overlying the patient.
► Follow-up abdominal CT (performed because of the history of trauma) and upright radiograph confirm the small pneumothorax (black arrows in Fig. 2.2 and 2.3).

Differential Diagnosis

► Deep sulcus sign of a left pneumothorax and a right pleural effusion are the two main considerations.

Teaching Points

► Because the most nondependent portion of the pleural space is at the base, a pneumothorax may be largest at the base on a supine radiograph. The base of the affected hemothorax may be more lucent and the costophrenic angle more apparent (deep sulcus sign).
► Care should be made to avoid confusion with blunting of the contralateral costophrenic angle from a pleural effusion on the other side.
► In patients on positive end-expiratory pressure mechanical ventilation (PEEP), a deep sulcus may prompt thoracostomy tube placement because of the potential for conversion to a larger pneumothorax.

Management

► Upright radiographs and decubitus films (side of suspected pneumothorax up) can be used to confirm that the deep sulcus is secondary to a pneumothorax.
► Although placement of a thoracostomy tube depends on clinical status, communication with the clinical team is essential because the deep sulcus sign is often quite subtle and often overlooked if images are viewed outside of a reading room.

Further Reading

Gordon R. The deep sulcus sign. *Radiology*. 1980 Jul;136(1):25-27.

History

▶ 42-year-old woman with shortness of breath receives this chest radiograph.

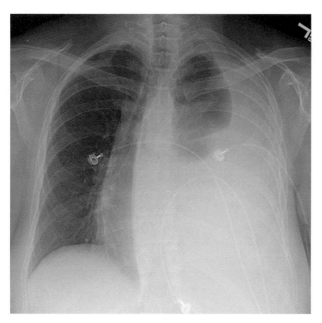

Figure 3.1

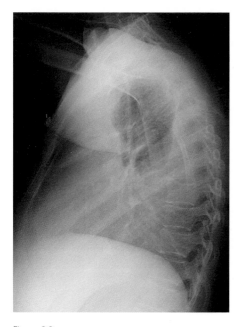

Figure 3.2

Case 3   Unilateral Pleural Effusion (Malignant)

Figure 3.3

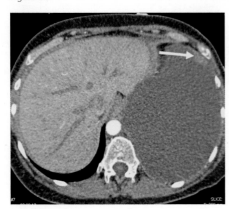

Figure 3.4

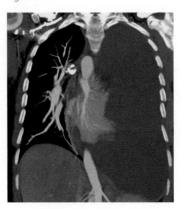

Findings

▶ Two-view chest radiograph (Figs. 3.1 and 3.2) shows increased opacification of the lower and lateral left hemothorax with a meniscus.

▶ The mediastinum is shifted rightward and the diaphragm is shifted inferiorly. The mass effect is better seen on the subsequent CT (Figs. 3.3 and 3.4). A small nodule is seen along the anterior pleura (arrow in Fig. 3.3).

Differential Diagnosis

▶ Unilateral pleural effusions are usually seen in infection (empyema), malignancy, and trauma (hemothorax). An abdominal process may present with a large unilateral effusion, such as a large right effusion in the setting of cirrhosis (hepatic hydrothorax). Other less common causes of large unilateral effusions include chylothorax, and glucothorax (from an extravascular placement of a central venous catheter).

Teaching Points

▶ Large unilateral effusions are rare in the setting of congestive heart failure and should prompt consideration of other potential etiologies.

▶ A large effusion may exert tension on surrounding structures and may have the same physiologic significance as a tension pneumothorax.

▶ A decubitus radiograph (side of effusion down) will show that the effusion is mobile when the effusion is small or medium. In larger effusions, there may be little appreciable change on a decubitus film.

Management

▶ Effusions under tension require drainage on an urgent/emergent basis.

▶ If the patient is hemodynamically stable, a CT may be performed for further characterization and thoracostomy tube planning.

Further Reading

Johnson JL. Pleural effusions in cardiovascular disease. Pearls for correlating the evidence with the cause. *Postgrad Med.* 2000 Apr;107(4):95-101.

History

▶ 21-year-old man with chest pain and shortness of breath after being shot in the back is imaged in the trauma suite.

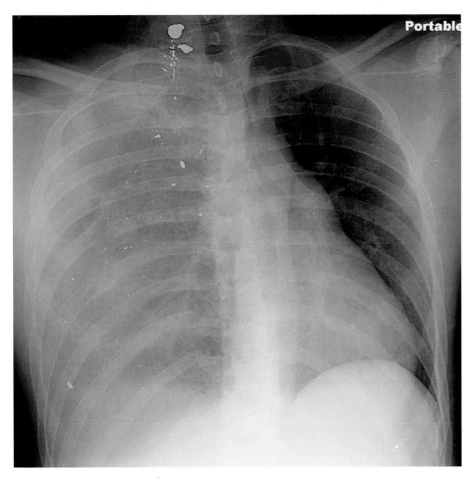

Figure 4.1

Case 4   Large Right Tension Hemopneumothorax

Figure 4.2

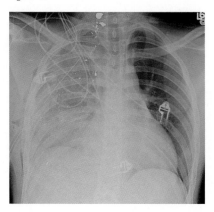

Findings

► Single-view portable radiograph shows multiple bullet fragments on the right with shift of the heart and mediastinum leftward. Pulmonary contusions and lacerations are seen near the bullet fragments.
► Increased opacification is seen in the right apex and increased lucency in the right base (Fig. 4.1).
► The tension component resolves after thoracostomy tube drainage (Fig. 4.2).

Differential Diagnosis

► Although the tension component may prompt one to consider pneumothorax, the density of the pleura is somewhat mixed. The combination of pleural densities is indicative of either a tension hydropneumothorax or a tension hemopneumothorax.

Teaching Points

► Hemopneumothorax usually follows trauma and can result in tension physiology. Penetrating trauma is more likely to result in a tension hemopneumothorax than blunt trauma.
► The radiographic appearance can be confusing because the presence of blood increases the attenuation of the pleural space.
► When supine, the fluid should collect in the more dependent location (apex) while the gas component will rise in the least dependent portion (base).

Management

► Tension hemopneumothorax requires emergent drainage.
► Further imaging is performed after thoracostomy tube drainage. The quantity and rate of drainage will help determine management. If the initial drainage is a large volume of blood or the rate of drainage is brisk, thoracotomy may be indicated.

Further Reading

Shanmuganathan K, Matsumoto J. Imaging of penetrating chest trauma. *Radiol Clin North Am*. 2006 Mar;44(2):225-238.

History

▶ 43-year-old woman with a history of omental carcinomatosis from an unknown primary tumor is admitted for increasing shortness of breath.

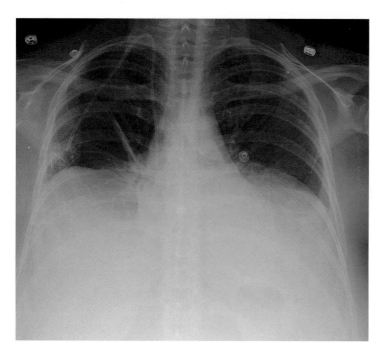

Figure 5.1

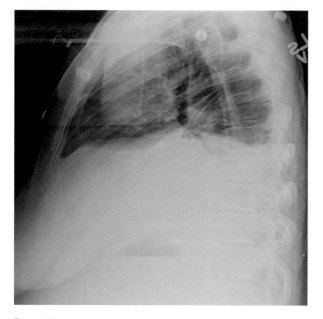

Figure 5.2

Case 5 Bilateral Subpulmonic Pleural Effusions

Figure 5.3

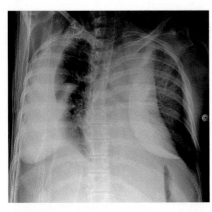

Figure 5.4

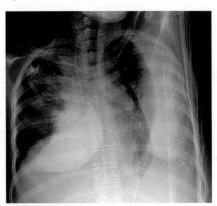

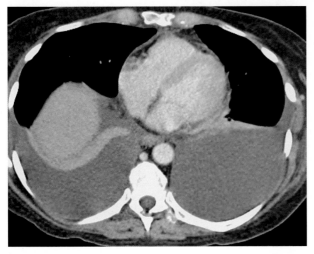

Figure 5.5

Findings

- ► Frontal radiograph (Fig. 5.1) shows increased distance between the stomach bubble and the left aerated lower lung. The right diaphragmatic peak is displaced lateral to the midclavicular line.
- ► On the lateral projection (Fig. 5.2), the posterior sulci are blunted, in keeping with pleural effusions.
- ► The large sizes of the pleural effusions are better appreciated on the bilateral decubitus films (Figs. 5.3 and 5.4) and the subsequent CT (Fig. 5.5).

Differential Diagnosis

- ► Bilateral large subpulmonic effusions and small lung volumes with elevated hemidiaphragms are the two main concerns.

Teaching Points

- ► When pleural fluid collects between the diaphragm and the lower lobe, it is referred to as a subpulmonic effusion.
- ► A subpulmonic effusion can be very hard to appreciate on an upright frontal radiograph. Findings of a subpulmonic effusion include increased distance between the stomach bubble and the left lung base (over 2 cm) and lateral displacement of the diaphragmatic peak on either side.

- Another sign of a subpulmonic effusion is the lack of visualization of pulmonary vessels below the dome of the diaphragm on the frontal radiograph.
- On the lateral radiograph, some degree of blunting of the posterior sulci is seen. Other findings include a horizontal contour to the diaphragm and fluid partially tracking up the oblique or major fissure (the thorn sign).
- Decubitus films can be performed to confirm the suspicion of the pleural effusion with the fluid layering on the dependent side. The lung parenchyma on the contralateral side can be simultaneously evaluated for an underlying pneumonia. (In this case no underlying pneumonia was seen.)
- A least 175 mL of fluid are required to cause blunting of the costophrenic angles on an upright film. The lateral decubitus is far more sensitive, detecting as little as 10 mL of fluid if done properly.

Management

- The management of a pleural effusion depends on the nature of the effusion and the clinical symptoms.
- An effusion under tension may require emergent drainage similar to a tension pneumothorax.
- An infected pleural effusion (an empyema) and hemothorax require drainage to prevent the development of a fibrothorax and trapped lung.

Further Reading

Yataco JC, Dweik RA. Pleural effusions: evaluation and management. *Cleve Clin J Med.* 2005 Oct;72(10):854-864.

History

▶ 22-year-old man complains of severe sudden onset of chest pain.

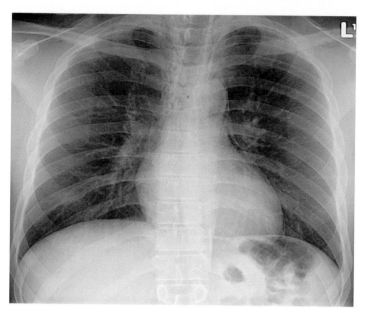

Figure 6.1

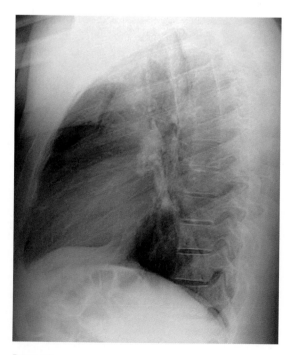

Figure 6.2

Case 6 Spontaneous Pneumomediastinum

Figure 6.3

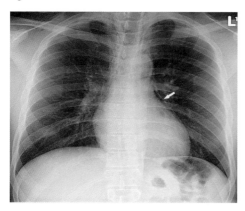

Figure 6.4

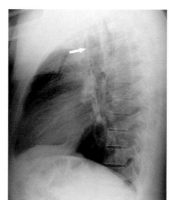

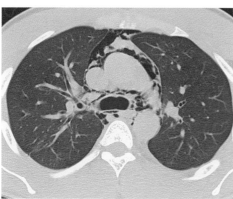

Figure 6.5

Findings

▶ Chest radiograph shows lucency adjacent to the left heart border (arrow in Fig. 6.3) on the frontal radiograph. Increased lucency is also seen around the aortic arch and in the right paratracheal region.
▶ On the lateral radiograph, the anterior wall of the trachea is very well seen (arrow in Fig. 6.4). Gas is also seen anterior to the ascending aorta.
▶ CT (Fig. 6.5) confirms the presence of gas centrally without fluid or evidence of tracheal rupture.

Differential Diagnosis

▶ Gas adjacent to the left heart border may be from pneumomediastinum, left pneumothorax, or pneumopericardium.

Teaching Points

▶ The internal webs (multiple radiopaque lines) are more typical of pneumomediastinum.
▶ Extension above the aortic arch, right paratracheal lucency, and subcutaneous gas are all seen with pneumomediastinum and not pneumopericardium.
▶ Pneumomediastinum may follow increased thoracic pressure from Valsalva or barotrauma.
▶ One may see pulmonary interstitial emphysema (PIE) or gas around the pulmonary vessels and bronchi when the etiology is barotrauma.
▶ Pneumomediastinum may also follow perforation of a hollow viscus (trachea, pharynx, or esophagus). Occasionally, pneumomediastinum may follow pneumoretroperitoneum or perforated bowel.

- Named signs of pneumomediastinum include a continuous diaphragm sign (when the entire diaphragm is seen on the frontal projection); the ring around the artery sign (gas around the extrapericardial pulmonary artery on a lateral projection); and the V of Naclerio (when the gas around the descending artery intersects the gas above the left hemidiaphragm behind the heart).
- Gas between the fascicles of the pectoralis major, also known as the gingko leaf sign, can occasionally be seen.
- Pneumomediastinum will not change appearance with decubitus images; however, pneumopericardium and pneumothorax will rise to the nondependent side.
- Pneumomediastinum may result in a pneumothorax, but pneumothorax should not result in a pneumomediastinum.

Management

- Because pneumomediastinum may be a finding of a ruptured viscus, management is often based on excluding tracheal, pharyngeal, or esophageal rupture. Endoscopy or a fluoroscopic esophageal study may be performed.
- Usually, spontaneous pneumomediastinum resolves in a few days without any intervention.

Further Reading
Bejvan SM, Godwin JD. Pneumomediastinum: old signs and new signs. *AJR Am J Roentgenol*. 1996 May;166(5):1041-1048.

History

▶ 26-year-old woman presents with sudden onset of chest and shoulder pain.

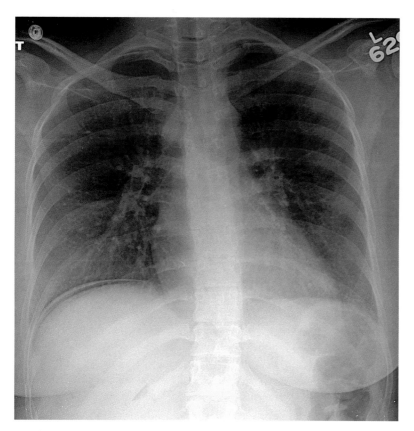

Figure 7.1

Case 7   Pneumoperitoneum (from a Perforated Ulcer)

Figure 7.2

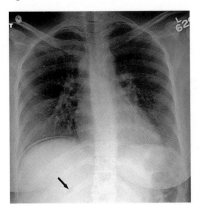

Findings

▶ Chest radiograph shows a crescentic lucency below the right hemidiaphragm (Fig. 7.1).

▶ Another lucency is seen above the right kidney (arrow in Fig. 7.2). This gas within the hepatorenal fossa has been called the "Doge's cap" sign, as it is said to resemble the headgear of the former leaders of Venice.

Differential Diagnosis

▶ Curvilinear lucency at the level of the right hemidiaphragm may represent either a subpulmonic pneumothorax or free intraperitoneal gas.

Teaching Points

▶ Because the differential includes both free intraperitoneal gas and pneumothorax, knowledge of the patient's position is key. On an upright study, gas in this location is most likely from free intraperitoneal gas. On a supine radiograph, the gas could be from either. An upright or left lateral decubitus film might be useful, as the pneumothorax is best seen at the apex (on the upright) or lateral aspect of the lung (on a contralateral decubitus).

▶ Care must be taken to exclude mimics of free intraperitoneal gas, including colonic interposition, in which haustra may be seen below the hemidiaphragm.

▶ Signs of pneumoperitoneum on chest radiography include curvilinear lucency beneath the hemidiaphragm, gas outlining the right border of the liver on a left lateral decubitus, Doge's cap, continuous diaphragm sign, and generalized increased lucency overlying the liver.

▶ Other signs, such as the Rigler sign (gas outlining both sides of bowel wall) and the triangle sign (gas within the mesentery between loops of bowel), may be seen.

▶ Pneumoperitoneum may follow intraperitoneal abdominal surgery or trauma, percutaneous catheter placement, or perforation of bowel. Less commonly, pneumoperitoneum may follow pneumomediastinum.

Management

▶ Because pneumoperitoneum may be a finding of a ruptured viscus, management is directed towards documenting its presence and excluding certain benign causes.

▶ When encountered in the reading room, one must look for any antecedent surgery or intervention. As a general rule, free gas should resolve by 7 to 10 days after surgery and decrease with time.

▶ Increasingly, CT is used to document pneumoperitoneum and reveal a potential source.

Further Reading

Chiu YH, Chen JD, Tiu CM, et al. Reappraisal of radiographic signs of pneumoperitoneum at emergency department. *Am J Emerg Med.* 2009 Mar;27(3):320-327.

History

▶ 72-year-old woman with a history of a mitochondrial myopathy receives this portable chest radiograph.

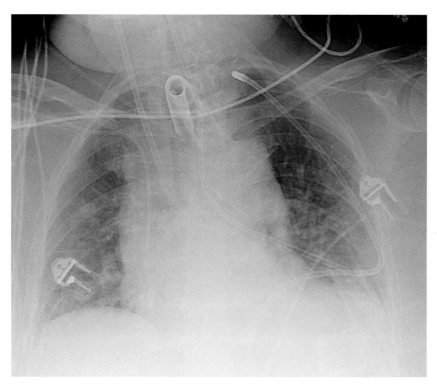

Figure 8.1

Case 8   Misplaced (Intrapleural) Nasogastric Tube

Figure 8.2

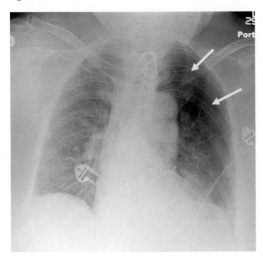

Findings

▶ Portable radiograph from the intensive care unit (ICU) (Fig. 8.1) shows a tracheostomy and right subclavian central line in usual position. The nasogastric tube, however, is not in the expected location. It can be seen entering the left mainstem bronchus and exiting the anteromedial basal segment into the pleural space, eventually ending up in the apex of the left hemithorax.

Differential Diagnosis

▶ There should be no differential diagnosis for the misplaced nasogastric tube.

Teaching Points

▶ Complications from misplaced feeding tubes are easily detected by chest radiography.
▶ Pleuropulmonary complications represent the most common complications after coiled feeding tubes in the pharynx/hypopharynx and placement in the distal esophagus. They result from inadvertent passage of tubes in the tracheobronchial tree with eventual perforation into the lung and pleural space.
▶ Because of the orientation of the bronchi, right bronchial placement is more common than left.
▶ Traditional clinical criteria of proper tube placement, including insufflation of air with sounds auscultated in the region of the stomach; aspiration of gastric fluid; and absence of cough, have been shown to be unreliable in ICU patients.

Management

▶ Obviously, a misplaced nasogastric tube should not be used for feeding. It should be removed. When communicating the finding to the ICU team, a follow-up radiograph should be suggested as these misplaced catheters may result in pneumothorax (arrows in Fig. 8.2).

Further Reading

Bankier AA, Wiesmayr MN, Henk C, et al. Radiographic detection of intrabronchial malpositions of nasogastric tubes and subsequent complications in intensive care unit patients. *Intensive Care Med.* 1997;23(4):406-410.
Lo JO, Wu V, Reh D, et al. Diagnosis and management of a misplaced nasogastric tube into the pulmonary pleura. *Arch Otolaryngol Head Neck Surg.* 2008 May;134(5):547-550.

History

▶ 66-year-old man with end-stage renal disease on dialysis reports decreased venous flow from his dialysis catheter.

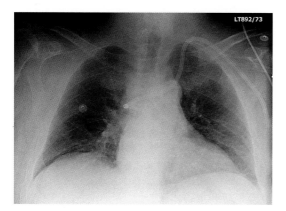

Figure 9.1

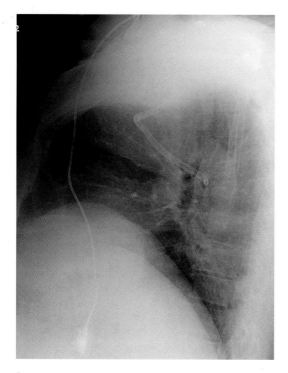

Figure 9.2

Case 9   Dialysis Catheter in the Azygos Vein

Figure 9.3

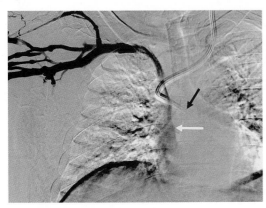

Figure 9.4

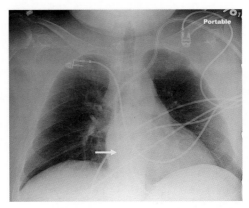

Findings
▶ Chest radiograph shows a left internal jugular dialysis catheter with a bend just above the right mainstem bronchus (Fig. 9.1). On the lateral radiograph (Fig. 9.2), the catheter heads posteriorly.
▶ The patient received a fistulogram that opacified the superior vena cava (white arrow in Fig. 9.3) and the catheter (black arrow in Fig. 9.3). The catheter was then redirected into the superior vena cava (white arrow in Fig. 9.4).

Differential Diagnosis
▶ Assuming the catheter has venous return, there should be no differential for the catheter location.

Teaching Points
▶ The azygos vein drains into the superior vena cava adjacent to the trachea just above the right mainstem bronchus.
▶ Although intentional placement of a central catheter into the azygos vein is a recognized endpoint in patients with severe venous occlusion, the azygos vein is not preferred for larger-bore dialysis catheters because of its relatively small caliber and direction of blood flow (away from the heart).
▶ Risk factors for azygos placement include left internal jugular venous access, catheters with long venous tips, and catheter insertion in a patient with fluid overload, where the azygous vein will be distended.
▶ The catheter in this case shows the path of the azygos vein on the chest radiograph. When distended, it can emulate right paratracheal lymphadenopathy on the frontal radiograph. The lateral view will show the distended vessel coursing behind the trachea (unlike lymphadenopathy, which is usually seen anterior to the trachea).

Management
▶ Management will depend on the type of device placed into the azygos vein.
▶ A hemodialysis catheter in the azygos vein runs the risk of venous perforation or thrombosis. For these reasons, larger-bore catheters are usually not kept in this location.
▶ However, purposeful placement of a defibrillator lead into the azygos can be used in the management of patients with elevated defibrillation threshold. In these cases, a lead ending in the azygos vein is the desired endpoint.

Further Reading
Bankier AA, Mallek R, Wiesmayr MN, et al. Azygos arch cannulation by central venous catheters: radiographic detection of malposition and subsequent complications. *J Thorac Imaging.* 1997;12:64-69.

History

▶ 84-year-old man with enterococcal bacteremia in need of intravenous antibiotics receives this radiograph to evaluate the location of the peripherally inserted central catheter.

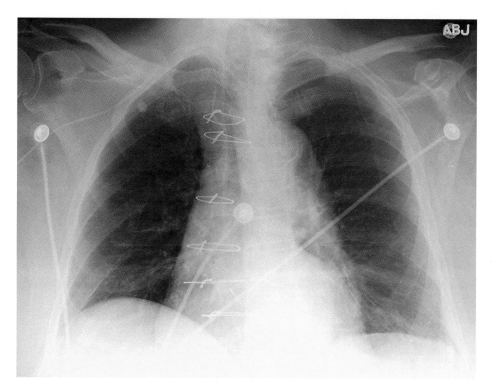

Figure 10.1

Case 10 Intraarterial (Subclavian Artery) Catheter Placement

Figure 10.2

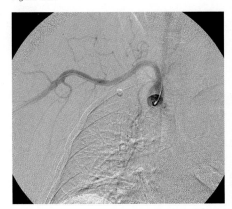

Figure 10.3

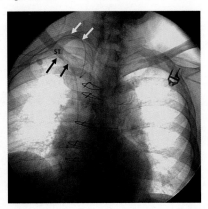

Findings

▶ Post-procedure radiograph (Fig. 10.1) shows a catheter coursing over the right apex and ending near the first sternal wire.

▶ Follow-up angiogram confirms the arterial course (Fig. 10.2). A new venous catheter was placed at the time of the angiogram (black arrows in Fig. 10.3). Note the difference in course compared to the arterial catheter (white arrows in Fig. 10.3).

Differential Diagnosis

▶ Arterial placement of the catheter should be the main consideration.

Teaching Points

▶ The subclavian vein passes anterior and inferior to the scalene tubercle (ST in Figure 10.3). Catheters within the vein are more horizontal than arterial catheters as they pass over the first rib. They then take a vertical course and point to the right atrium.

▶ Subclavian arterial catheters pass superior and posterior to the scalene tubercle and follow the apical margin of the lung. They point towards the aorta, or the innominate artery.

▶ Arterial placement is a rare complication. Usually it is without consequence, but it may lead to life-threatening complication if a large-bore dilator or catheter is inserted.

▶ Arterial placement may follow a direct puncture but also may follow a transvenous puncture, in the setting of a fistula.

▶ If arterial placement is suspected, a blood gas can be sent for analysis to distinguish venous from arterial blood. Another option is to connect the line to a pressure transducer to see whether an arterial or venous wave form is present.

Management

▶ If an arterial placement is suspected, the line should not be pulled without seeking consultation from a vascular surgeon.

▶ If arterial injury with a large-caliber catheter occurs, prompt surgical treatment seems to be the safest approach. The pull followed by pressure technique is often associated with risk of hematoma, airway obstruction, stroke, or false aneurysm.

Further Reading

Guilbert MC, Elkouri S, Bracco D, et al. Arterial trauma during central venous catheter insertion: Case series, review and proposed algorithm. *J Vasc Surg.* 2008 Oct;48(4):918-925.

Nicholson T, Ettles D, Robinson G. Managing inadvertent arterial catheterization during central venous access procedures. *Cardiovasc Intervent Radiol.* 2004 Jan-Feb;27(1):21-25.

History

▶ 28-year-old man with a history of myasthenia gravis is noted to be hypoxic.

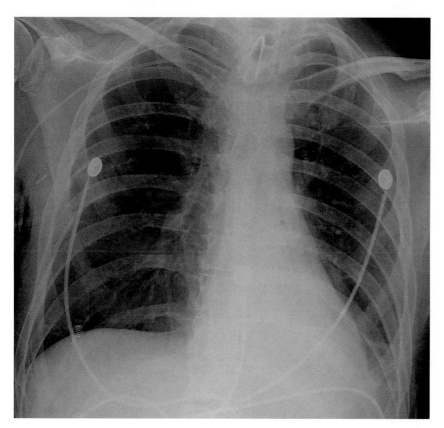

Figure 11.1

Case 11   Left Lower Collapse (from a Mucus Plug)

Figure 11.2

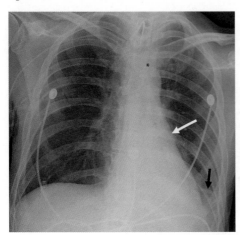

Figure 11.3

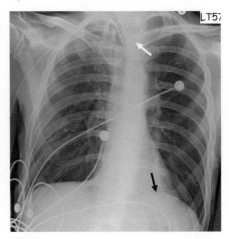

Findings

▶ Initial chest radiograph (Fig. 11.1) shows a retrocardiac opacity with air bronchograms and narrowed distances between the left ribs. The left hemidiaphragm cannot be seen behind the heart and the left heart border appears straightened. Also note the inferior location of the left hilum.

▶ Follow-up chest radiograph obtained the following day shows near-complete resolution. The left hemidiaphragm can now be seen (black arrow in Fig. 11.3) and the left heart border has regained the normal curvature. The peripherally inserted catheter flipped into the left brachiocephalic vein (white arrow in Fig. 11.3).

Differential Diagnosis

▶ Left lower lobe collapse and pneumonia are the two main considerations. The volume loss strongly supports the former.

Teaching Points

▶ Left lower lobe collapse assumes the shape of a left retrocardiac triangle. The base of the triangle will obscure the left hemidiaphragm.

▶ The aerated upper lobe will allow the left heart border to be visible. The volume loss results in leftward rotation of the heart. The net result is an altered appearance to the cardiac silhouette more akin to a right anterior oblique projection.

▶ The altered left heart border appears straighter than normal. This finding has been referred to as the flat waist sign (white arrow in Fig. 11.2).

▶ Lingular linear atelectasis is another finding in left lower lobe collapse (Nordentsrom's sign). This comes from the altered orientation of the lingular bronchi with hyperexpansion (black arrow in Fig. 11.2).

▶ Two other findings of left lower lobe collapse include shift of the anterior junction line and the top of the knob sign. In the latter, shifted mediastinal soft tissues obscure the top of the aortic arch (asterisk in Fig. 11.2).

Management

▶ With simple collapse, management rests on pulmonary toilet and occasional bronchoscopy to clear the mucus. If no prior studies are available, the collapse should be followed to resolution to exclude a central mass.

Further Reading

Gurney JW. Atypical manifestations of pulmonary atelectasis. *J Thorac Imaging.* 1996 Summer;11(3):165-175.
Woodring JH, Reed JC. Radiographic manifestations of lobar atelectasis. *J Thorac Imaging.* 1996 Spring;11(2):109-144.

History

▶ 69-year-old woman is admitted for hemoptysis.

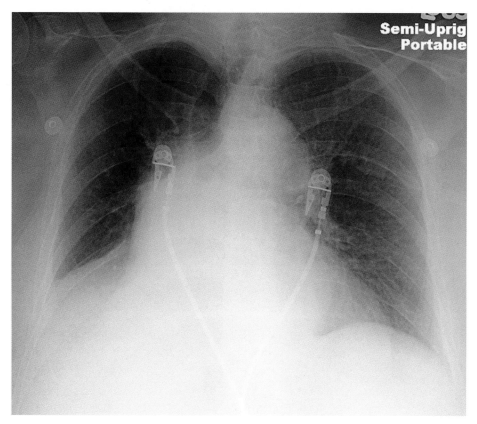

Figure 12.1

Case 12 Right Middle Lobe and Right Lower Collapse (from Central Bronchogenic Carcinoma)

Figure 12.2

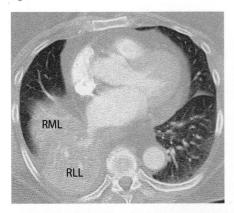

Figure 12.3

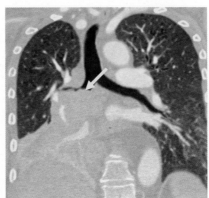

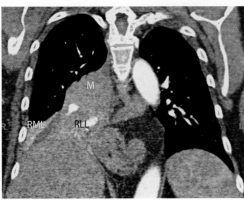

Figure 12.4

Findings

► On the initial radiograph (Fig. 12.1), the right heart border and hemidiaphragm are obscured.
► Associated volume loss is noted, which can best be seen by the rightward shift of the heart and mediastinum.
► CT was performed the next day, which showed the collapsed lobes (Fig. 12.2; RML = middle lobe and RLL = right lower lobe). Reconstructions more clearly delineate the central mass (white arrow in Fig. 12.3) and the collapsed lobes (RML = middle lobe, RLL = lower lobe, and m = mass in Fig. 12.4).

Differential Diagnosis

► Based on the radiograph, right middle lobe and right lower lobe collapse should be the main consideration.

Teaching Points

► Right middle and lower lobe collapse is the result of obstruction of the bronchus intermedius, from either mucus or an endobronchial lesion.
► The volume loss of both lobes results in inferior displacement of the minor and major fissures. Usually, the minor fissure falls below the level of the major fissure and the major fissure extends superiorly to the hilum (see Fig. 12.4). The net composite is the "S-shaped" opacity as seen above, especially when a central mass is present.

- Right middle and lower lobe collapse displaces the right hilum inferiorly and obscures the descending right interlobar artery.
- Shift of the heart and mediastinum rightward is frequently seen with this combination of collapse.
- To prevent confusion with a right pleural effusion, one must remember that an effusion is higher laterally and combined right middle and lower lobe collapse is higher medially.
- The double lesion sign refers to collapse of two segments that are not in proximity. Because of the anatomic distance, a single lesion (cancer) is not plausible. An example of the double lesion sign would include right upper and lower lobe collapse without middle lobe involvement.

Management

- With simple collapse, the management rests on pulmonary toilet and occasional bronchoscopy to clear the mucus. Collapse should be compared to a prior study or followed to resolution to exclude a central mass.

Further Reading

Woodring JH, Reed JC. Radiographic manifestations of lobar atelectasis. *J Thorac Imaging.* 1996 Spring;11(2):109-144.

History

▶ 62-year-old woman with a 2-month history of a nonproductive cough receives this chest radiograph.

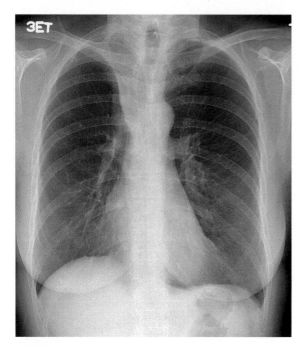

Figure 13.1

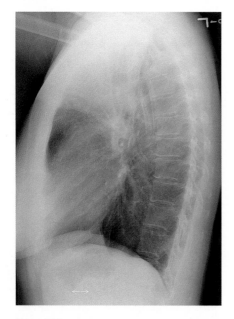

Figure 13.2

Case 13 Right Upper Lobe Collapse with a Reverse S of Golden (from an Endobronchial Carcinoid Tumor)

Figure 13.3

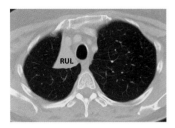

Figure 13.4

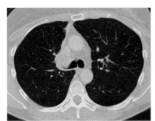

Figure 13.5

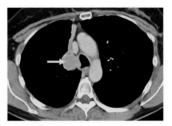

Findings

▶ Chest radiograph shows volume loss on the right with an elevated right hemidiaphragm and right hilum. Right paratracheal opacity is seen in keeping with right upper lobe collapse. The interface with the lung approximates the shape of a reverse S and has come to be known as the (reverse) S sign of Golden. Note the very faint juxtaphrenic peak.

▶ Follow-up CT confirmed the right upper lobe collapse (RUL in Fig. 13.3) and central mass (arrow in Fig. 13.5). This mass obstructs the right upper lobe bronchus and is hyperenhancing. As would be expected, this was a carcinoid tumor.

Differential Diagnosis

▶ Based on the radiograph, the two main concerns would be right upper lobe collapse from a mass or bland right upper lobe collapse.

Teaching Points

▶ Right upper lobe collapse may be from mucus plugging, peripheral airways disease (such as tuberculosis), or an endobronchial lesion.

▶ The presence of a central mass creates an inferior bulge that helps create an inverse S between the collapsed lung and the aerated lung.

▶ Other findings of right upper lobe collapse include a juxtaphrenic peak in which either an inferior accessory fissure or the inferior pulmonary ligament pulls on the hemidiaphragm (akin to marionette strings), an elevated right hilum, and findings of volume loss.

▶ Rarely, right upper lobe collapse has been associated with a pneumothorax that is thought to result from a vacuum phenomenon. Akin to a joint vacuum phenomenon, this type of pneumothorax has come to be known as a pneumothorax *ex vacuo*. This pneumothorax will dissipate only if the central mass is cleared. It will not resolve with thoracostomy drainage.

▶ When right upper lobe collapse is combined with right middle lobe collapse, malignancy should strongly be considered.

Management

▶ With simple collapse, the management rests on pulmonary toilet and occasional bronchoscopy to clear the mucus. The collapse should be compared with prior images or followed to resolution to exclude an underlying mass.

Further Reading

Woodring JH, Reed JC. Radiographic manifestations of lobar atelectasis. *J Thorac Imaging*. 1996 Spring;11(2):109-144.

History

▸ 28-year-old woman with asthma comes to the Emergency Department with worsening dyspnea.

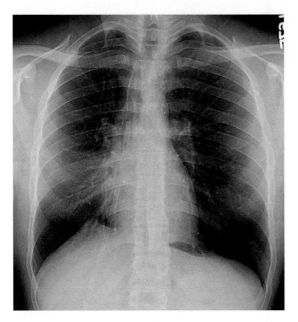

Figure 14.1

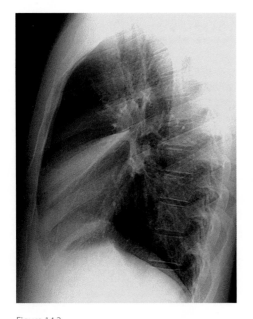

Figure 14.2

Case 14 Right Middle Lobe Collapse (from a Mucus Plug)

Figure 14.3

Figure 14.4

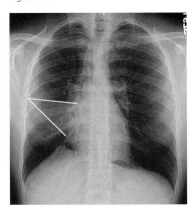
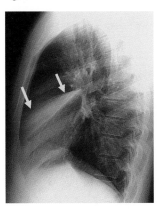

Findings

► Initial frontal radiograph (Fig. 14.1) contains a vague triangular opacity that effaces the right heart border (overlay in Fig. 14.3). Accompanying volume loss is best appreciated by the effect on the right hemidiaphragm.
► On the lateral radiograph (Fig. 14.2), the lobar collapse is seen as a dense triangle with a central apex and the base against the anterior chest wall. The superior border is made up by the horizontal (minor) fissure (arrows in Fig. 14.4) and the inferior edge by the major fissure. The orientation of the minor fissure explains why it is no longer clearly seen on the frontal radiograph.

Differential Diagnosis

► Right middle lobe collapse and right middle lobe consolidation from pneumonia are the two main considerations. The volume loss strongly supports the former.

Teaching Points

► Right middle lobe collapse is the lobar collapse least associated with volume loss as it is the lobe with the least volume.
► Early collapse is associated with effacement of the right heart border known as the silhouette sign.
► As the collapse progresses, it pulls the minor fissure inferiorly out of the transverse plane. The net effect is that the minor fissure is no longer well seen on the frontal projection.
► The lateral radiograph is characteristic for right middle lobe collapse. The volume loss results in approximation of the major and minor fissures with a resultant dense triangle over the heart.
► Rarely, right middle lobe collapse may be longstanding as a result of chronic inflammation, bronchiectasis, or fibrosis. The term *right middle lobe syndrome* has been used to refer to chronic nonobstructive, right middle lobe collapse.

Management

► With simple collapse, the management rests on pulmonary toilet and occasional bronchoscopy to clear the mucus.
► With a central mass, the treatment is aimed towards diagnosing the mass, usually by bronchoscopic biopsy, and then surgical resection, if possible.

Further Reading

Gurney JW. Atypical manifestations of pulmonary atelectasis. *J Thorac Imaging.* 1996 Summer;11(3):165-175.
Woodring JH, Reed JC. Radiographic manifestations of lobar atelectasis. *J Thorac Imaging.* 1996 Spring;11(2):109-144.

History

▶ 53-year-old woman with increasing shortness of breath presents with worsening cough.

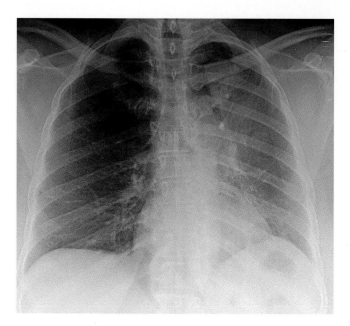

Figure 15.1

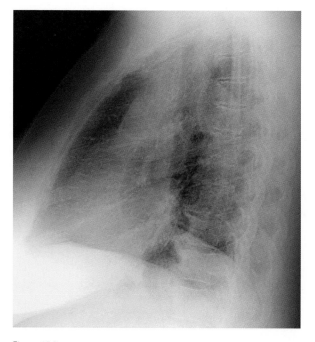

Figure 15.2

Case 15   Left Upper Lobe Collapse (from a Non-Small Cell Lung Cancer)

Figure 15.3

Figure 15.4

Figure 15.5

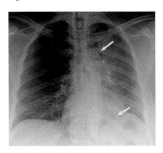 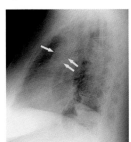 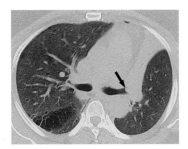

Findings

► Increased lucency around the aortic arch (Luftsichel sign) (superior arrow in Fig. 15.3) with vague area of increased opacity in the left upper lobe on the frontal radiograph.
► Volume loss is seen on the left with mild elevation of the left hemidiaphragm and questionable juxtaphrenic peak (inferior arrow in Fig. 15.3).
► On the lateral projection, opacity is seen overlying the ascending aorta with increased retrosternal clear space representing the hyperexpanded right lung (single arrow in Fig. 15.4).
► CT confirms the findings and shows the endobronchial mass (arrow in Fig. 15.5).

Differential Diagnosis

► Left upper lobe collapse, probably from a mass. There should be no differential diagnosis.

Teaching Points

► Left upper lobe collapse can be the hardest lobar collapse (atelectasis) to diagnose on chest radiography.
► Plain film findings on the frontal radiograph include a vague left upper lobe opacity, increased lucency around the aortic knob (Luftsichel sign) that represents the hyperexpanded left lower lobe, left volume loss, and a left juxtaphrenic peak.
► On the lateral radiograph one may see an anterior opacity bordered by the oblique fissure and hyperexpanded lower lobe posteriorly (double arrow in Fig. 15.4) and the hyperexpanded right lung anteriorly (single arrow in Fig 15.4).

Management

► Though rarely mucus may result in left upper lobe collapse, most causes of pure upper lobe collapse are from an endobronchial mass. For this reason, when encountered on a chest radiograph, left upper lobe collapse usually prompts a CT and then bronchoscopy. In this case, the mass was found to be a squamous cell carcinoma by bronchoscopic biopsy.

Further Reading

Proto AV. Lobar collapse: basic concepts. *Eur J Radiol.* 1996 Aug;23(1):9-22.
Woodring JH, Reed JC. Radiographic manifestations of lobar atelectasis. *J Thorac Imaging.* 1996 Spring;11(2):109-144.

History

▶ 25-year-old woman with a long history of tobacco use presents with fever and cough.

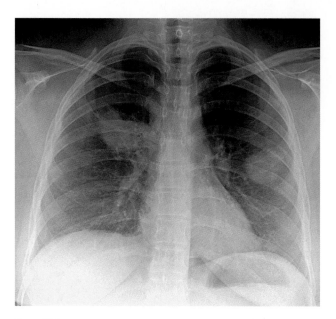

Figure 16.1

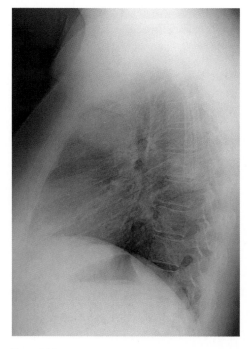

Figure 16.2

Case 16 Bilateral Round Pneumonia (Community-Acquired)

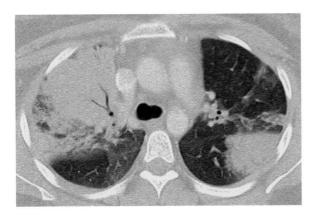

Figure 16.3

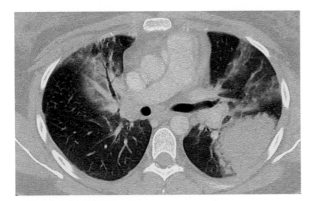

Figure 16.4

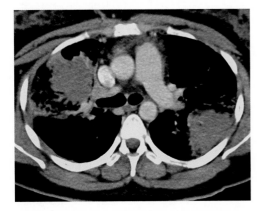

Figure 16.5

Findings

▶ Chest radiograph (Figs. 16.1 and 16.2) shows bilateral mass-like opacities with mild right paratracheal lymphadenopathy and no pleural effusions.

▶ CT (Figs. 16.3, 16.4, and 16.5) performed the next day clearly delineates the air bronchograms within the opacities. On the CT, the consolidation in the right upper lobe has taken more of a lobar pneumonia pattern.

Differential Diagnosis

▶ For bilateral masses on a chest radiograph, the differential diagnosis would be headed by neoplasm or infection. Less likely would be congenital lesions such as pulmonary arteriovenous malformations. Care must be taken on viewing an initial radiograph, as occasionally community-acquired pneumonia may present with such a tumefactive appearance. Comparison with old studies is key in getting this diagnosis right.

Teaching Points

▶ Community-acquired pneumonias tend to be symptomatic on presentation with fever and cough.

▶ Of the community-acquired pneumonias, *Streptococcus pneumoniae* is the organism most often associated with a round pneumonia.

▶ Cavitation is rare and effusions are seen in less than 50% of patients with round pneumonia.

▶ Pneumonia often has air bronchograms for two reasons: the pus-filled airspaces serve as a natural contrast for the air-filled bronchi, and the adjacent inflammation results in mild bronchial dilatation (akin to an ileus when inflammation surrounds a bowel loop, as in pancreatitis). These dilated bronchi do not represent bronchiectasis as they are not permanently dilated.

Management

▶ Any airspace process requires comparison of the current film with a prior one to determine acuity and to prevent confusion for a mass.

▶ Usually, the patient will be treated for community-acquired pneumonia with antibiotics. The pneumonia should clear in 2 weeks, as it did here.

▶ In older patients or in those with atypical clinical manifestations, radiography will be performed to document resolution. This is performed to prevent overlooking a neoplasm, such as lymphoma or bronchioloalveolar carcinoma, that may manifest as airspace disease.

Further Reading

Franquet T. Imaging of pneumonia: trends and algorithms. *Eur Respir J.* 2001 Jul;18(1):196-208.

History

▶ 46-year-old woman with worsening dyspnea on exertion presents to the Emergency Department.

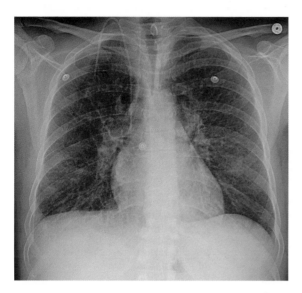

Figure 17.1

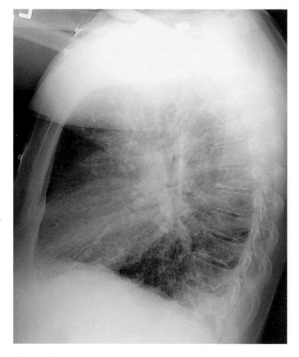

Figure 17.2

Case 17 Congestive Heart Failure

Figure 17.3

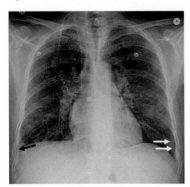

Figure 17.4

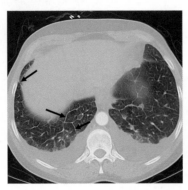

Figure 17.5

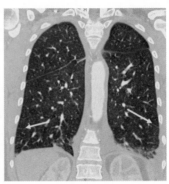

Findings

▶ Chest radiograph (Figs. 17.1 and 17.2) shows small effusions and interstitial opacities that can be followed to the pleural surface. These horizontal, thickened interlobular septae are referred to as *Kerley B lines* (white arrows in Fig. 17.3).

▶ CT confirmed the findings of pulmonary edema with small pleural effusions. Note the smooth interlobular septal thickening (black arrows in Fig. 17.4 and white arrows in Fig. 17.5).

▶ Small pleural effusions can also be seen (black arrow in Fig. 17.3).

Differential Diagnosis

▶ Before launching into a differential diagnosis of interstitial disease, comparison should be made to any prior studies. Once we know this is an acute process, edema versus atypical pneumonia (viral) are favored.

Teaching Points

▶ Pulmonary edema can be classified as hydrostatic (cardiogenic) or from increased vascular permeability (noncardiogenic).

▶ Hydrostatic edema may be from cardiac causes (decreased left ventricular function, mitral/aortic valve disease), pulmonary venous obstruction, fluid overload (renal failure), or hypoalbuminemia.

▶ Noncardiogenic edema or edema from increased permeability is less likely to present with Kerley B lines.

▶ Edema with increased permeability may be seen in a variety of conditions, including inhalation injuries, trauma, high altitude, shock, drugs, and neurologic disease.

▶ Edema from a mixed hydrostatic increased permeability pattern may be seen in neurogenic edema, high-altitude edema, re-expansion edema, postsurgery edema, or illicit drugs (crack, cocaine).

▶ Radiograph findings of cardiogenic pulmonary edema include subpleural edema (seen as fissural thickening), pleural effusions, and interlobular septal line thickening.

▶ Other findings of cardiogenic edema include pulmonary vascular redistribution, peribronchial cuffing, and lack of visualization of the hilar vessels. Often, the heart is mildly enlarged. Occasionally, consolidation may be present.

Management

▶ Management is based on severity of the pulmonary edema.

▶ Unilateral edema may prompt a CT to exclude an underlying central mass (fibrosing mediastinitis or lung cancer).

Further Reading

Webb WR. Pulmonary edema. The acute respiratory distress syndrome, and radiology in the intensive care unit. In Webb WR, Higgins CB, eds. *Thoracic Imaging: Pulmonary and Cardiovascular Radiology*. Philadelphia: Lippincott Williams and Wilkins, 2005:330-335.

History

► 28-year-old woman is admitted for severe back pain. Because of fever, a chest radiograph was obtained.

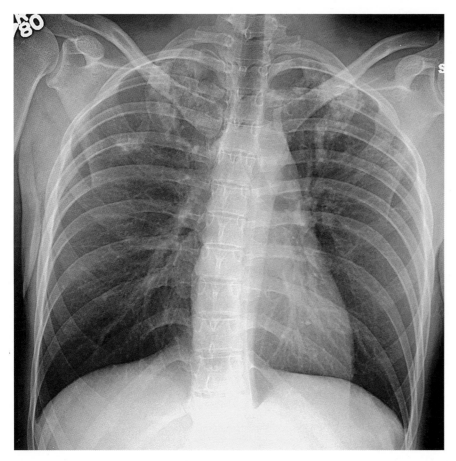

Figure 18.1

Case 18   Active Tuberculosis

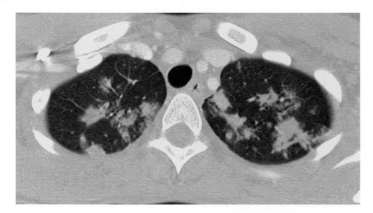

Figure 18.2

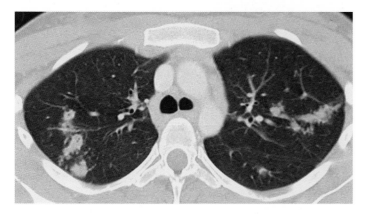

Figure 18.3

Findings

▶ Initial radiograph (Fig. 18.1) shows bilateral upper lung reticulonodular airspace disease without pleural effusions or lymphadenopathy.

▶ CT (Figs. 18.2 and 18.3) confirms the nodules. Some of these abut the pleura. CT confirmed the absence of lymphadenopathy or pleural effusions.

Differential Diagnosis

▶ The differential diagnosis is based on the upper lobe predominance. Practically, it includes cystic fibrosis, sarcoidosis, pulmonary Langerhans cell histiocytosis, and tuberculosis (TB). In a young patient with fever, TB must be considered first.

Teaching Points

▶ TB is a common infection in the developing world and in certain pockets in the United States.

▶ Transmission is by aerosolized particles that are highly resistant to dehydration, water, or alcohol. TB easily spreads in contained environments with poor ventilation, such as prisons, schools, nursing homes, or hospitals.

▶ The primary site of infection, known as the *Ghon focus*, usually presents with lymphadenopathy (especially in children) and spontaneously heals. The Ghon focus may result in consolidation in any lobe of the lungs.

- The *Ranke complex* refers to the combination of the Ghon focus and the lymphadenopathy.
- Pleural effusions may be seen in primary infection.
- Healed primary infection usually results in a calcified granuloma. The mycobacteria are not always cleared from these granulomata.
- In 5% to 10% of patients, endogenous reactivation of TB occurs years after the primary infection. This postprimary TB is usually seen in the apical and posterior segments of the upper lobes and the superior segments of the lower lobes.
- Effusions are unusual with postprimary TB and lymphadenopathy is typically absent.
- Postprimary TB usually presents with poorly defined nodules and may cavitate.
- In postprimary TB, endobronchial dissemination may manifest with a tree-in-bud appearance. Hematogenous spread results in miliary nodules.
- DNA analysis has challenged the traditional classification of TB into primary versus postprimary based on chest radiography. The radiographic appearance seems to be more dependent on host immunity.

Management

- Once TB is suspected, the patient must be placed in respiratory isolation and sputum should be sent to stain for the acid-fast bacilli and for culture.

Further Reading

Jeong YJ, Lee KS. Pulmonary tuberculosis: up-to-date imaging and management. *AJR Am J Roentgenol.* 2008 Sep;191(3):834-844.

History

▶ 15-month-old boy is admitted for new-onset wheezing.

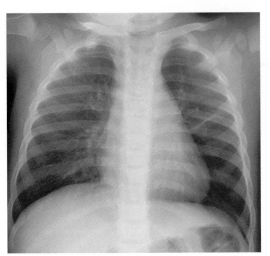

Figure 19.1

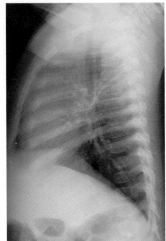

Figure 19.2

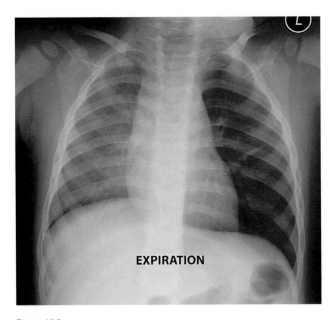

Figure 19.3

Case 19 Aspirated Foreign Body (Peanut in Left Mainstem Bronchus)

Findings

▶ The admission chest radiographs (Figs. 19.1 and 19.2) are deceptively near-normal in their appearance. There may be minimal hyperlucency to the left lung, which is normal in size.

▶ The expiration image clearly demonstrates air-trapping in the left lung (Fig. 19.3).

Differential Diagnosis

▶ The differential diagnosis based on a lucent lung with air-trapping would include Swyer-James-Macleod syndrome, endobronchial foreign body, congenital lobar overinflation, and aspirated foreign body.

▶ Swyer-James-Macleod usually results in a smaller lung with air-trapping and does not present with acute wheezing. Congenital lobar overinflation should be localized to one lobe (usually the left upper lobe) and should have mass effect on the normal lung.

Teaching Points

▶ Most aspirated foreign bodies are radiolucent on radiography.

▶ Most foreign body aspirations are seen in children younger than 10 years.

▶ Medications, ethanol, and illicit drug use can increase the likelihood of aspiration in older patients.

▶ Radiographic suggestion of radiolucent aspirated foreign body requires demonstration of air trapping or collapse.

▶ Air-trapping can be demonstrated by failure of a lung or part of the lung to collapse during expiration imaging. If the patient is too young to follow commands, a radiograph or fluoroscopic image can be obtained during crying. Alternatively, decubitus views can be obtained. The lung with the endobronchial foreign body will not collapse when it is the side placed down.

▶ Most foreign bodies are aspirated into the lower lobes. Because of the vertical nature of the bronchus intermedius, the right lower lobe is a more common site than the left lower lobe.

▶ Vegetable matter is one of the more common aspirated materials. Over time, a radiolucent endobronchial foreign body may calcify.

Management

▶ Aspirated foreign bodies should be removed. Their presence can elicit proliferation of granulation tissue, which predisposes to recurrent or chronic pneumonias, stenosis, bronchiectasis, or hemoptysis.

▶ Endobronchial foreign bodies are usually removed bronchoscopically. Very rarely, when the foreign body has been present for a long period of time, lobectomy is required.

Further Reading
Shepard JA. The bronchi: an imaging perspective. *J Thorac Imag.* 1995;10:236-254.

History

▶ 86-year-old man is admitted with dyspnea and fatigue.

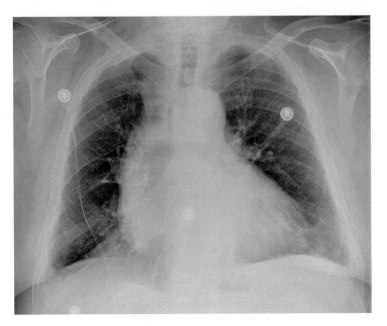

Figure 20.1

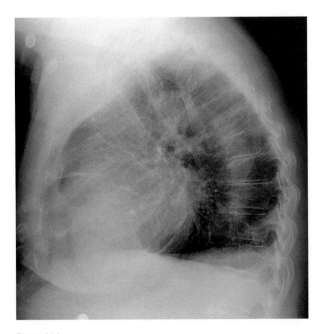

Figure 20.2

Case 20   Pericardial Effusion with Fat Pad (Sandwich) Sign

Figure 20.3

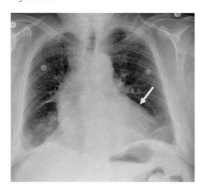

Figure 20.4

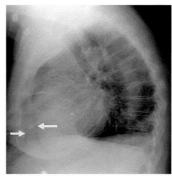

Figure 20.5

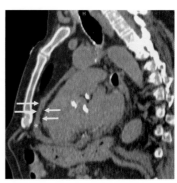

Findings

▶ Initial radiograph (Figs. 20.1 and 20.2) shows global enlargement of the cardiac silhouette without pulmonary vascular redistribution or pulmonary edema. On the frontal, the cardiac silhouette is less dense along the left heart border (differential density sign) (arrow in Fig. 20.3).

▶ On the lateral view, two radiolucent arcs can be seen near the anterior chest wall (arrows in Fig. 20.4). These represent the epicardial and pericardial fat separated by pericardial fluid. This finding has been referred to as the fat pad sign, sandwich sign, or Oreo cookie sign. CT reconstruction (Fig. 20.5; asterisk = pericardial fluid; anterior arrows = pericardial fat; posterior arrows = epicardial fat) shows how the fat pads can create this sign.

Differential Diagnosis

▶ Dilated cardiomyopathy or pericardial effusion can explain an enlarged cardiac silhouette without pulmonary edema or vascular redistribution. The presence of the sandwich sign confirms the latter.

Teaching Points

▶ Sonography is used for the initial detection and characterization of pericardial effusions.

▶ Although the water bottle appearance of the heart is well published, the ability to detect this configuration prospectively is somewhat limited.

▶ When global enlargement of the cardiac silhouette is encountered, comparison should be made to prior radiographs. Sudden changes in cardiac size should prompt one to consider pericardial effusion over cardiomyopathy.

▶ The differential density sign refers to decreased attenuation of the cardiac periphery from a pericardial effusion. As no heart is in this portion, the pericardial fluid attenuates the x-ray beam less than the central portion.

▶ On the lateral radiograph, the fat pad sign may be seen. Normally the pericardial stripe should be only 2 to 4 mm.

▶ Pericardial effusions may be secondary to collagen vascular diseases (especially lupus), myxedema, uremia, radiation, and infection (viral or mycobacterial). Occasionally, they may be malignant or sanguineous (hemopericardium).

Management

▶ The initial finding of global enlargement of the cardiac silhouette on a chest radiograph should prompt an echocardiogram.

▶ Management is based on the size of the effusion and its effect on the heart.

Further Reading

Woodring JH. The lateral chest radiograph in the detection of pericardial effusion: a reevaluation. *J Ky Med Assoc.* 1998 Jun;96(6): 218-224.

Part 2   Congenital Lesions

History

▶ 64-year-old female smoker had an abnormality detected on preoperative chest radiograph prior to knee replacement surgery.

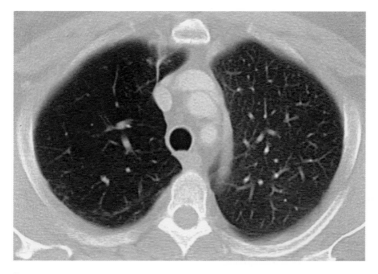

Figure 21.1

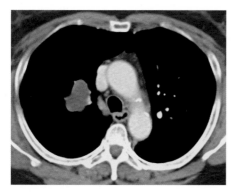

Figure 21.2

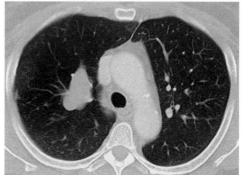

Figure 21.3

Case 21 Bronchial Atresia

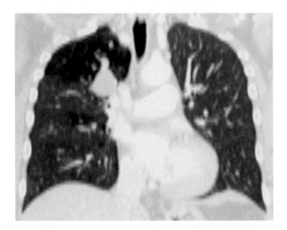

Figure 21.4

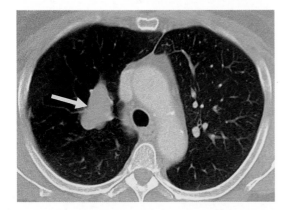

Figure 21.5

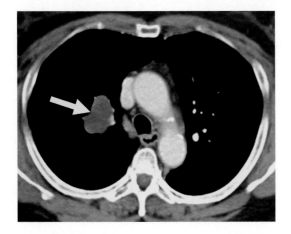

Figure 21.6

Findings

▸ A smoothly marginated, low-attenuation branching opacity (arrows in Figs. 21.5–21.6) is noted in the right upper lobe (mucocele).

▸ Hyperlucency, indicative of air trapping, is noted in the right upper lobe peripheral to the central tubular opacity.

Differential Diagnosis

▸ In this case, the features are pathognomonic of bronchial atresia (air-trapping with low-attenuating, central branching mass).

Teaching Points

▸ Resulting from atresia of a central bronchus, most commonly a segmental bronchus, bronchial atresia is likely the result of airway maldevelopment or potentially an *in utero* vascular insult.

▸ A mucus-impacted bronchus (mucocele) and surrounding lung hyperinflation, due to collateral air drift, are pathognomonic findings on CT.

▸ Close scrutiny of the central airway to exclude an endobronchial mass (such as carcinoid or squamous cell carcinoma) is recommended, as these masses can occasionally present with distal air-trapping.

Management

▸ The majority of cases are incidental findings on studies performed for other reasons and require no further follow-up or management. A small percentage of cases can present with recurrent infections, which may necessitate surgical resection.

Further Reading

Gipson MG, Cummings KW, Hurth KM. Bronchial atresia. *Radiographics*. 2009 Sep-Oct;29(5):1531-1535.

Martinez S, Heyneman LE, McAdams HP, et al. Mucoid impactions: finger-in-glove sign and other CT and radiographic features. *Radiographics*. 2008 Sep-Oct;28(5):1369-1382.

History

▶ 68-year-old woman with epistaxis receives this chest CT without and with intravenous contrast.

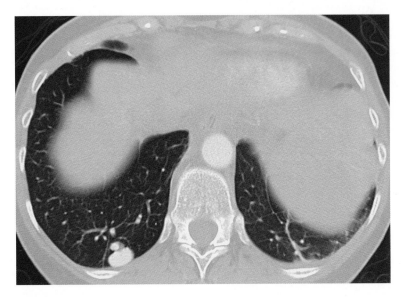

Figure 22.1

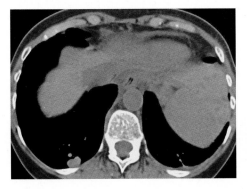

Figure 22.2

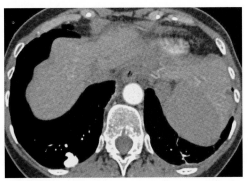

Figure 22.3

Case 22   Pulmonary Arteriovenous Malformation (AVM) (in Hereditary Hemorrhagic Telangiectasia)

Figure 22.4

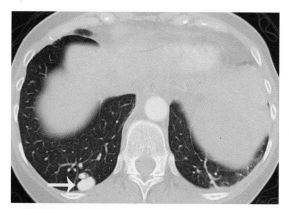

Figure 22.5

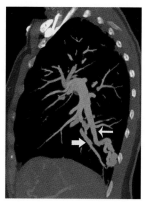

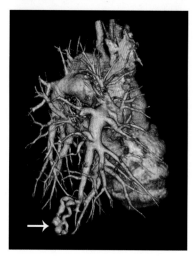

Figure 22.6

Findings

▶ Avid contrast enhancement of a smoothly marginated pulmonary nodule in the right lower lobe is seen (arrow in Fig. 22.4).

▶ Sagittal maximum intensity projection image demonstrates a single large feeding artery (small arrow in Fig. 22.5) and draining vein (thick arrow in Fig. 22.5). These findings are confirmed on the volume-rendered image, which nicely shows the AVM (arrow in Fig. 22.6).

Differential Diagnosis

▶ The main differential for a very high-attenuating nodule on CT includes a pulmonary AVM, granuloma, carcinoid tumor, or vascular metastasis. Once the feeding artery and draining vein are seen, the diagnosis is made. Occasionally a pulmonary varix can simulate an AVM in the setting of fibrosing mediastinitis. No feeding artery should be seen with a varix.

Teaching Points

▶ Nearly 80% of patients with a pulmonary AVM will have underlying hereditary hemorrhagic telangiectasia (HHT), an autosomal dominant disorder.

▶ Due to right-to-left shunting, patients with HHT and pulmonary AVMs can suffer from hypoxia, stroke, or brain abscesses. When numerous, they can even present with hypoxia.

▶ Recurrent epistaxis is a common presenting symptom for patients with HHT.

▶ Another group of patients at risk for the development of AVM are those with congenital heart disease treated with cavopulmonary anastomoses, presumably due to absence of exposure to a hepatic angiogenesis inhibitor.

▶ Multi-detector CT pulmonary angiography is now used for screening in patients with HHT. Multiplanar reconstructions to demonstrate the feeding artery(ies) and draining vein(s) are useful adjuncts to the transverse images.

Management

▶ The most important information regarding management is the size of the feeding pulmonary artery, measured near the nidus, not the nidus size itself. AVMs with feeding arteries 3 mm or greater are treated with coil embolization.

▶ If HHT is suspected, referral to a subspecialty center is recommended for appropriate management and screening of relatives.

Further Reading

Cottin V, Dupuis-Girod S, Lesca G, Cordier JF. Pulmonary vascular manifestations of hereditary hemorrhagic telangiectasia (Rendu-Osler Disease). *Respiration.* 2007;74(4):361-378.

Cummings KW, Bhalla S. Multidetector computed tomographic pulmonary angiography: Beyond acute pulmonary embolism. *Radiol Clin North Am.* 2010 Jan;48(1):51-65.

History

▶ 35-year-old man with progressive shortness of breath undergoes a chest CT.

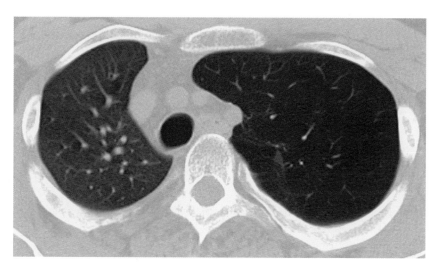

Figure 23.1

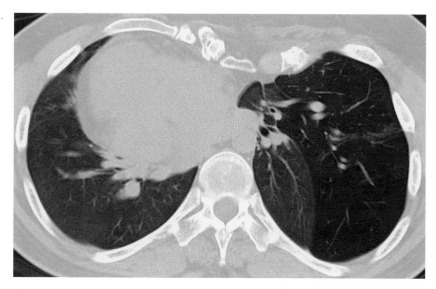

Figure 23.2

Case 23   Congenital Lobar Hyperinflation (Emphysema)

Figure 23.3

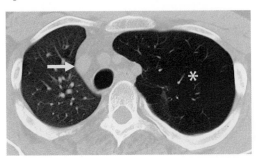

Figure 23.4

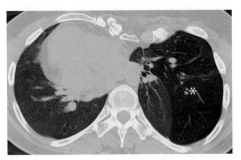

Findings

► Hyperlucency (asterisk in Fig. 23.3) in the left upper lobe is indicative of marked air-trapping.

► Mass effect of the hyperinflated left upper lobe causes mediastinal shift rightward (arrow in Fig. 23.3) and compresses the left lower lobe (asterisk in Fig. 23.3 and 23.4).

Differential Diagnosis

► Congenital lobar hyperinflation or central obstructing lesion/foreign body could both explain the mass effect and air-trapping. Given lack of central mass, the former is favored.

Teaching Points

► Congenital lobar hyperinflation reflects airspace enlargement, not destruction as seen in emphysema. Hence, the term *congenital lobar hyperinflation* is preferred over *congenital lobar emphysema*.

► This condition can result from intrinsic (bronchomalacia, webs, stenoses) or extrinsic (compression by adjacent vascular structures, bronchogenic cysts) causes affecting the central airways.

► While Swyer-James syndrome, an acquired obliterative bronchiolitis presumably due to prior infection, also causes air-trapping accentuated on exhalation sequences, the affected lung is smaller and does not exert mass effect.

Management

► Symptoms related to compression of adjacent structures or lobes may necessitate surgical lobectomy, as in this case.

Further Reading

Berrocal T., Madrid C., Novo S., et al. Congenital anomalies of the tracheobronchial tree, lung and mediastinum: embryology, radiology, and pathology. *Radiographics*. 2004 Jan-Feb;*24*(1):e17.

History

▶ 60-year-old woman with shortness of breath and abnormal chest radiograph undergoes subsequent CT.

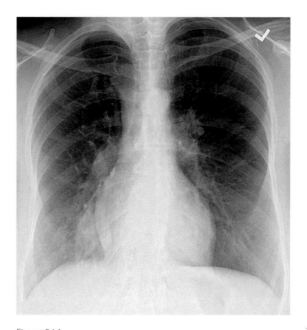

Figure 24.1

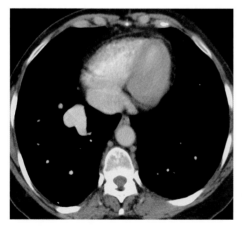

Figure 24.2

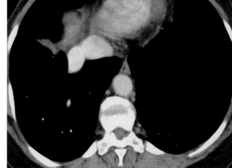

Figure 24.3

Case 24 Hypogenetic Venolobar Syndrome (Scimitar Syndrome)

Figure 24.4

Figure 24.5

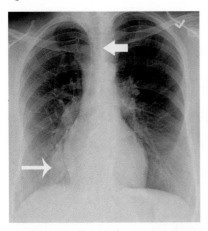

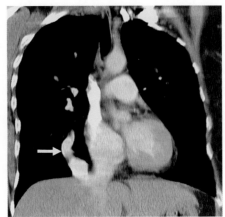

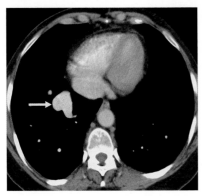

Figure 24.6

Findings

▶ Tubular opacity (thin arrow in Fig. 24.4) courses lateral to the right heart border in the right lung base. There is mild right hemithorax volume loss as evidenced by subtle mediastinal shift rightward (thick arrow in Fig. 24.4).

▶ CT demonstrates venous drainage from the right lung into a large tubular vein (arrows in Figs. 24.5 and 24.6) coursing to the inferior vena cava.

Differential Diagnosis

▶ Based on the chest radiograph alone, right lower lobe atelectasis, pneumonia, or mass lesions, including malignancy or sequestration, may be considered. Given the additional CT findings, congenital hypogenetic venolobar (or scimitar) syndrome is the diagnosis.

Teaching Points

▶ Almost always right-sided, scimitar syndrome reflects partial anomalous pulmonary venous drainage from the right lower lobe or entire lung to the systemic system, most commonly the inferior vena cava. There is associated underdevelopment of the right lung.

▶ Coexistent cardiac abnormalities, such as atrial septal defects, may also be present.

- Rarely, an anomalous systemic artery from the aorta may feed the right lower lung. This artery should not be confused with a sequestration.
- Meandering pulmonary veins, which take a tortuous course through the lung before eventually draining to the left atrium, can mimic scimitar veins, especially on a chest radiograph.

Management

- Longstanding left-to-right shunting can lead to pulmonary hypertension, requiring surgical correction of the partial anomalous venous return and any associated cardiac defects.
- The size of the shunt will determine whether the lesion will be repaired.

Further Reading

Ahamed MF, Al Hameed F. Hypogenetic lung syndrome in an adolescent: Imaging findings with a short review. *Ann Thorac Med*. 2008 Apr;3(2):60-63.

Zylak CJ, Eyler WR, Spizarny DL, Stone CH. Developmental lung anomalies in the adult: radiologic-pathologic correlation. *Radiographics*. 2002 Oct; 22 Spec No:S25-43.

History

▶ 55-year-old man with a new diagnosis of rectal cancer undergoes staging CT.

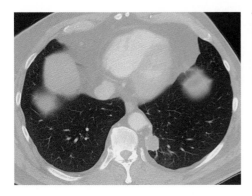

Figure 25.1

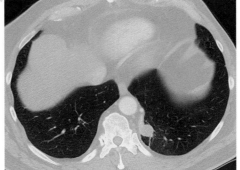

Figure 25.2

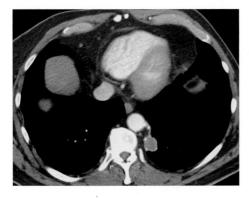

Figure 25.3

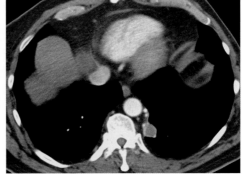

Figure 25.4

Case 25 Intralobar Sequestration

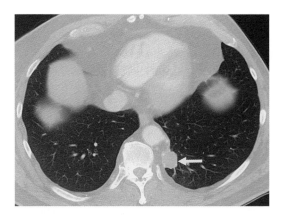

Figure 25.5

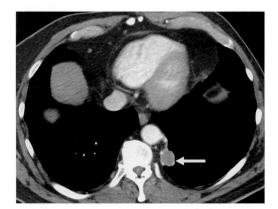

Figure 25.6

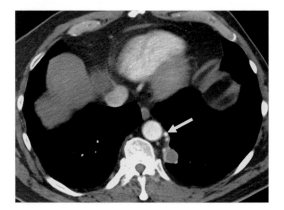

Figure 25.7

Findings

▶ CT images show a well-circumscribed low-attenuation nodule (arrows in Figs. 25.5 and 25.6) in the left lower lobe with systemic arterial feeders (arrow in Fig. 25.7) arising from the descending thoracic aorta.

Differential Diagnosis

▶ The identification of the nodule might raise the specter of metastasis but the low-attenuation, rounded nature of the lesion should make one consider a congenital lesion (sequestration, cystic adenomatoid malformation, or bronchogenic cyst), infectious lesion, or even a benign lesion, such as a hamartoma. Once the feeding vessels are seen, a sequestration is the only plausible diagnosis.

Teaching Points

▶ A sequestration comprises nonfunctioning pulmonary tissue in isolation from the tracheobronchial tree and has systemic arterial supply.
▶ Sequestrations may be divided into two categories: intralobar and extralobar. Intralobar sequestrations are more commonly seen in adults and share a pleural covering with the remainder of the lung. The feeding arteries tend to come from the descending thoracic aorta and the veins drain into the pulmonary veins or left atrium.
▶ Given overlap in histologic features with other congenital lung malformations, especially bronchial atresia, intralobar sequestrations may represent true congenital lesions, though many believe the lesion to be acquired, possibly due to recurrent infection.
▶ Extralobar sequestrations are less common in adults and actually have a distinct pleural envelope from the remainder of the lung. Their feeding arteries more commonly arise from the abdominal aorta or celiac axis and the veins drain into the systemic veins.
▶ Intralobar sequestrations can be cystic or solid and not uncommonly have surrounding air-trapping.

Management

▶ Usually these lesions are discovered incidentally, especially in adults; therefore, no further workup or intervention is needed. Occasionally, the lesions can become superinfected and require surgical resection.

Further Reading

Frazier AA, Rosado de Christenson ML, Stocker JT, Templeton PA. Intralobar sequestration: radiologic-pathologic correlation. *Radiographics*. 1997 May-Jun;17(3):725-745.
Langston C. New concepts in the pathology of congenital lung malformations. *Semin Pediatr Surg*. 2003 Feb;12(1):17-37.

History

▶ 16-year-old girl with asthma presents with this CT.

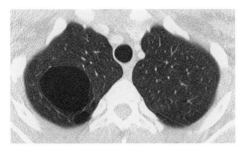

Figure 26.1

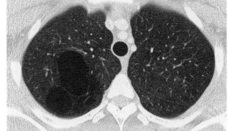

Figure 26.2

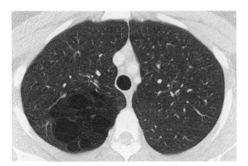

Figure 26.3

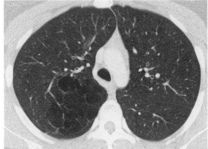

Figure 26.4

Case 26 Congenital Cystic Adenomatoid Malformation

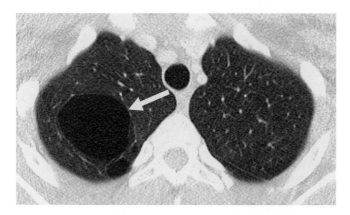

Figure 26.5

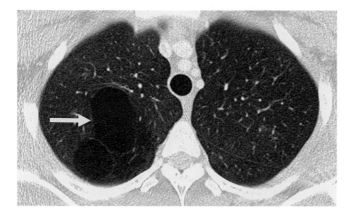

Figure 26.6

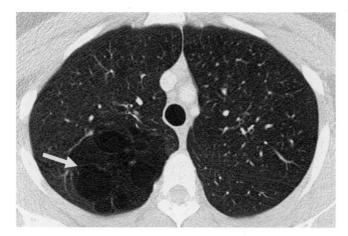

Figure 26.7

Findings

▶ CT demonstrates localized conglomeration of medium-sized and large cysts (arrows in Figs. 26.5-26.7) in the apical and posterior segments of the right upper lobe without adjacent airspace disease or pleural effusion.

Differential Diagnosis

▶ Based on the CT features, the differential consists of cystic adenomatoid malformation, cystic intralobar sequestration, or postinfectious pneumatoceles.

Teaching Points

▶ Cystic adenomatoid malformation is a congenital lesion with abnormal bronchiolar proliferation. The "cysts" are actually massively dilated bronchioles.

▶ The Stocker classification system divides these lesions into type I (large cysts >2 cm), type II (multiple small cysts <2 cm), and type III (solid, microcystic lesions). Type II and III lesions have been associated with a poor prognosis, probably from their frequent association with other congenital anomalies. Type I lesions do have a low likelihood of developing malignancies, such as bronchoalveolar carcinoma.

▶ The majority of lesions are detected in childhood as masses on chest radiographs in infants with respiratory distress. Initially, the lesion may appear solid, but over the first 24 to 48 hours of life fluid clears from the lesion, leaving cystic airspaces. In older children or adults, these lesions can be encountered incidentally or come to attention due to mass effect or superinfection.

Management

▶ In children, these lesions are routinely resected. In adults, lesions are resected if symptomatic, but do not necessarily require radiographic follow-up if asymptomatic.

Further Reading

Bush A. Congenital lung disease: a plea for clear thinking and clear nomenclature. *Pediatr Pulmonol.* 2001 Oct;32(4):328-337.

Epelman M, Kreiger PA, Servaes S, et al. Current imaging of prenatally diagnosed congenital lung lesions. *Semin Ultrasound CT MR.* 2010 Apr;31(2):141-157.

Part 3 Mediastinal Lesions

History

▶ 48-year-old woman with chest pain receives a CT, using the pulmonary embolism protocol. She was then referred for an MR of the chest.

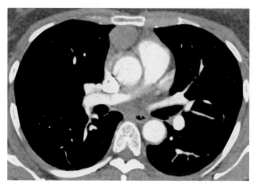

Figure 27.1

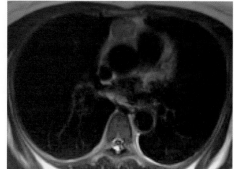

Figure 27.2

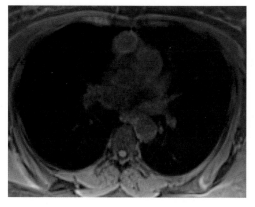

Figure 27.3

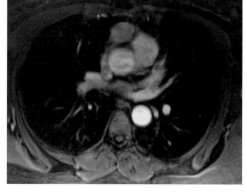

Figure 27.4

Case 27 (Noninvasive) Thymoma

Figure 27.5

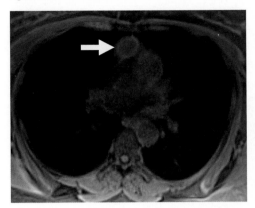

Figure 27.6

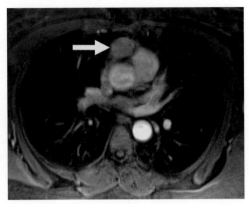

Findings

▶ CT (Fig. 27.1) shows an anterior mediastinal mass that measures 64 HU. Because of the potential for a complex thymic cyst, she was referred for MR.

▶ HASTE (Fig. 27.2), pre-contrast (Fig. 27.3), and post-gadolinum fat-saturated T1-weighted (Fig. 27.4) images demonstrate a homogenous, well-encapsulated, smoothly contoured mass (arrows in Figs. 27.5 and 27.6) with homogenous enhancement.

Differential Diagnosis

▶ In a 48-year-old woman with an incidental encapsulated, solid mass, the main differential diagnosis consists of lymphoma versus thymoma.

Teaching Points

▶ Thymoma is the most common neoplasm of the anterior mediastinum, usually affecting middle-aged and older adults. It is often an incidental finding, though rarely extrinsic compression may cause symptoms.

▶ The terms "invasive" and "noninvasive" are used instead of benign and malignant as invasive tumors may not show evidence of malignancy on pathology, but can be difficult to treat and aggressive. Imaging features indicative of invasion include mediastinal fat, vascular or lung invasion, and pleural-based metastases.

▶ MR can be useful in differentiating benign thymic conditions from neoplasms. Using fat suppression or chemical shift sequences, MR can differentiate the fatty composition of thymic hyperplasia from the more soft tissue composition of thymoma and lymphoma.

▶ MR can also be useful in confirming a thymic cyst. Pre- and post-contrast images will show lack of enhancement.

▶ Patients with thymoma have a 30% to 40% likelihood of having myasthenia gravis. A smaller percentage (10–15%) of patients with myasthenia gravis will have thymoma.

▶ Other parathymic associations in patients with thymoma include pure red cell aplasia and hypogammaglobulinemia.

Management

▶ Surgical excision is the treatment of choice, which in the setting of a noninvasive thymoma can often be accomplished transcervically, avoiding the need for median sternotomy.

Further Reading

Nishino M, Ashiku SK, Kocher ON, et al. The thymus: a comprehensive review. *Radiographics*. 2006;26:335-348.

Sadohara J, Fujimoto K, Muller NL, et al. Thymic epithelial tumors: comparison of CT and MR imaging findings of low-risk thymomas, high-risk thymomas, and thymic carcinomas. *Eur J Radiol*. 2006 Oct;60(1):70-79.

History

► 21-year-old man with exertional dyspnea is sent for a chest radiograph.

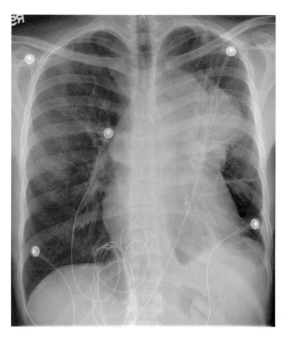

Figure 28.1

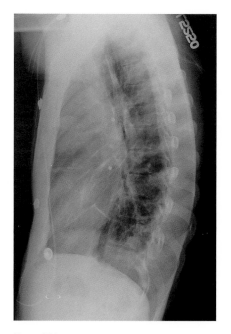

Figure 28.2

Case 28 Anterior Mediastinal Mass (Diffuse Large B-cell Lymphoma)

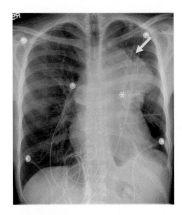

Figure 28.3

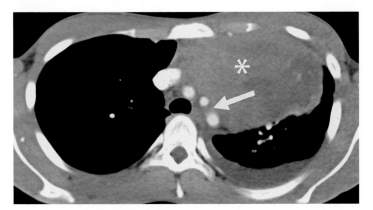

Figure 28.4

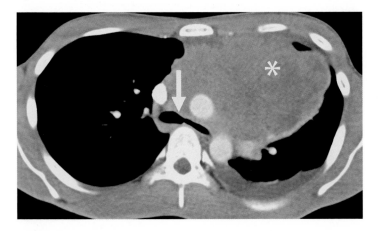

Figure 28.5

Findings

► On the frontal radiograph, a soft-tissue-density mass (arrow in Fig. 28.3) silhouettes the aortic arch and aorticopulmonary window. The left hilar vessels (asterisk in Fig. 28.3) can be seen through the mass (hilum overlay sign) and the descending thoracic aortic line is preserved.

► On the lateral, the mass fills in the retrosternal clear space. The trachea is also displaced posteriorly and compressed against the spine.

► CT images demonstrate a slightly heterogenous soft tissue mass (asterisk in Figs. 28.4 and 28.5) centered within the anterior mediastinum, encasing the great vessels (arrow in Fig. 28.4) and displacing the trachea and left mainstem bronchus posteriorly (arrow in Fig. 28.5).

Differential Diagnosis

► Because the mass is mostly soft tissue with only few areas of fluid attenuation, the differential diagnosis would include lymphoma, malignant germ cell tumor, and less likely thymic mass, such as thymoma.

Teaching Points

► The most commonly encountered anterior mediastinal masses in adults are thymoma and lymphoma. Germ cell tumors are more common in younger patients.

► While Hodgkin's lymphoma is the most common form presenting in the anterior mediastinum, diffuse large B-cell lymphomas have a propensity for the anterior mediastinum in young adults and can present with symptoms related to compression of vessels and the airway.

► Lymphomas of the mediastinum tend to surround vessels but rarely compress them. Occasionally, lymphomas extend anteriorly into the chest wall.

► The hilum overlay sign (lack of obscuration of the hilar structures [i.e. bronchi, pulmonary arteries and veins]) on plain radiograph indicates that a mass lies within the anterior or posterior mediastinum. When the posterior mediastinal lines, descending thoracic aortic stripe, and paravertebral lines are preserved, localization can be made to the anterior mediastinum.

Management

► If no easily accessible nodes, such as supraclavicular or axillary, are involved, many anterior mediastinal masses can be approached parasternally via CT or US guidance for tissue sampling. For lymphoma, fine-needle aspiration for flow cytometry and core biopsy should be performed.

Further Reading

Whitten CR, Khan S, Munneke GJ, Grubnic S. A diagnostic approach to mediastinal abnormalities. *Radiographics*. 2007 May-Jun;27(3): 657-671.

History

▸ 16-year-old boy with chest pain receives this CT after a motor vehicle collision.

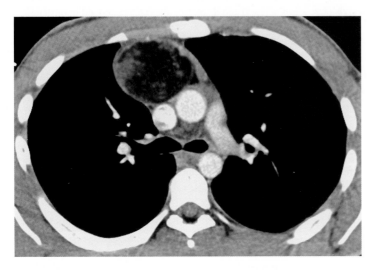

Figure 29.1

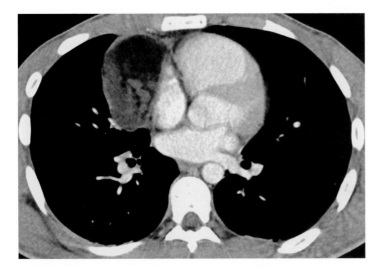

Figure 29.2

Case 29 Mature Teratoma

Figure 29.3

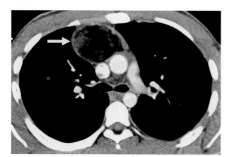

Figure 29.4

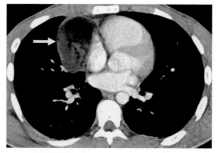

Findings

▶ Fat- and fluid-attenuation anterior mediastinal mass (arrows in Figs. 29.3 and 29.4) extends inferiorly along the right heart border.

Differential Diagnosis

▶ Because of the fat, the differential diagnosis would include teratoma (benign germ cell tumor), thymolipoma, and rarely liposarcoma. Given that fat is the dominant attenuation and there are few areas of fluid attenuation, teratoma should be favored.

Teaching Points

▶ Mature teratoma is the most common germ cell tumor of the mediastinum and affects the sexes relatively equally, coming to clinical attention most often incidentally.
▶ Teratomas arise near or within the thymus and are made up of various combinations and amounts of soft tissue, fat, and calcification. While infrequently seen, formed teeth or fat/fluid levels are considered diagnostic.
▶ While teratomas are considered benign, if components of other germ cell tumor lines are present they are more appropriately referred to as mixed germ cell tumors.
▶ The ratio of fluid/fat to soft tissue can be helpful in distinguishing between benign and malignant germ cell tumors. In benign lesions, the fat/fluid components are far greater than any soft tissue element.

Management

▶ Because of the mass effect and the very small chance of malignant elements, surgical excision is the treatment of choice.

Further Reading

Rosado-de-Christenson ML, Templeton PA, Moran CA. From the archives of AFIP. Mediastinal germ cell tumors: radiologic and pathologic correlation. *Radiographics*. 1992 Sep;12(5):1013-1030.

History

▶ 27-year-old man presenting with chest pain and fatigue is referred for chest CT.

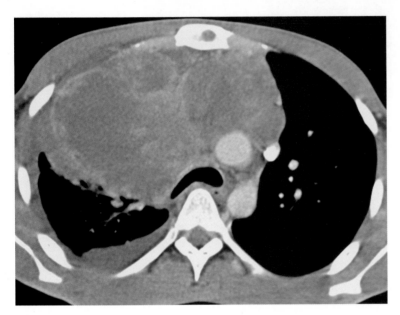

Figure 30.1

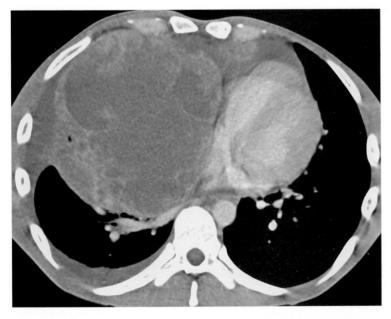

Figure 30.2

Case 30 Malignant Germ Cell Tumor (Primary Mediastinal Yolk Sac Tumor)

Figure 30.3

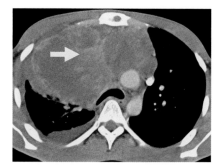

Figure 30.4

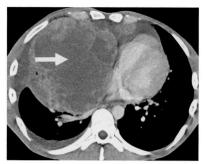

Findings

▶ Large heterogeneous soft tissue mass (arrows in Figs. 30.3 and 30.4) centered in the anterior mediastinum exerting posterior mass effect on the trachea and compressing the right cardiac chambers. Note how much soft tissue attenuation is present compared with the volume of fluid attenuation. In addition to the mass effect on the vessels, the superior vena cava is compressed and occluded.

Differential Diagnosis

▶ Because of the size of the lesion and its heterogeneity, the mass is most likely to be a malignant germ cell tumor or lymphoma. Rarely, sarcomas may present similarly.

Teaching Points

▶ Mediastinal germ cell tumors account for approximately 15% of anterior mediastinal masses in adults. Mature teratomas (see case 29), which may contain fat and calcification, are most common, with seminomas and nonseminomatous malignant germ cell tumors accounting for the remainder.

▶ While teratomas are seen in relatively equal frequency in both sexes, malignant germ cell tumors are seen more commonly in young male patients. The most common malignant germ cell tumor is a seminoma.

▶ Nonseminomatous malignant germ cell tumors include embryonal cell carcinoma, yolk sac tumors, choriocarcinomas, and mixed cell types. These tend to be grouped together because of their rarity and poor prognosis. They tend to look similar on CT imaging.

▶ Serologic tumor markers (LDH, alpha fetoprotein, beta-hCG) are tested and followed in nonseminomatous malignant germ cell tumors.

▶ While cystic changes can be seen in benign tumors, such as mature teratoma, a higher ratio of soft tissue to cystic change should raise concern for malignant tumors that have undergone necrosis, such as malignant germ cell tumors, sarcomas, or potentially treated metastases or lymphoma.

Management

▶ Percutaneous biopsy with CT or ultrasound guidance can frequently be used for tissue sampling, especially in larger masses. Remember to look for easily accessible nodal sites (supraclavicular or axillary) if there is metastatic adenopathy.

▶ Mature teratomas are surgically excised. Seminomatous germ cell tumors are treated with radiation with or without surgical resection. Nonseminomatous malignant germ cell tumors have the worst prognosis and are usually treated with chemotherapy and sometimes surgical resection.

Further Reading

Rosado-de-Christenson ML, Templeton PA, Moran CA. From the archives of AFIP. Mediastinal germ cell tumors: radiologic and pathologic correlation. *Radiographics*. 1992 Sep;12(5):1013-1030.

History

▶ 55-year-old man with chest discomfort receives this chest radiograph.

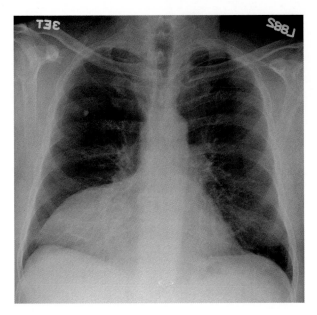

Figure 31.1

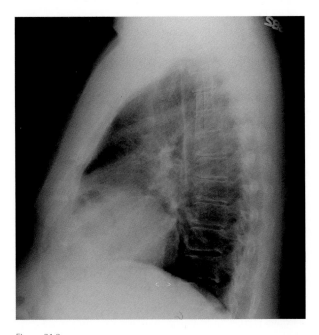

Figure 31.2

Case 31 Foramen of Morgagni Diaphragmatic Hernia

Figure 31.3

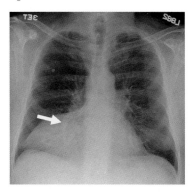

Figure 31.4

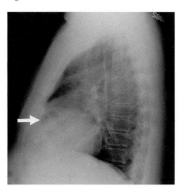

Findings

▸ Right cardiophrenic angle soft tissue mass is seen on the frontal radiograph, obscuring the right heart border. Right interlobar and lower lobe pulmonary arteries (arrow in Fig. 31.3) can still be seen (hilum overlay sign, suggesting anterior mediastinal process).

▸ On the lateral radiograph, the soft tissue mass is located anteriorly and contains a loop of partially air-filled bowel (arrow in Fig. 31.4).

Differential Diagnosis

▸ Foramen of Morgagni hernia, pericardial cyst, abundant pericardial fat, lymphadenopathy/lymphoma, or other anterior mediastinal mass (thymoma, germ cell tumor) should be considered when a right cardiophrenic angle mass is encountered. Identification of the bowel loop makes the foramen of Morgagni the most likely diagnosis.

Teaching Points

▸ Resulting from a defect in the attachment of diaphragmatic muscle fibers to the costal margin and central tendon of the diaphragm, foramen of Morgagni hernias are relatively rare (<3% diaphragmatic hernias).

▸ They are more commonly right-sided, and usually contain herniated omentum or portions of the transverse colon.

Management

▸ CT can be used to confirm the diagnosis and exclude other differential entities when the diagnosis is not clear on the radiograph. Herniation of omental fat into the retrosternal space is noted at CT and can be differentiated from abundant pericardial fat by omental vessels coursing through the fat or herniated abdominal viscera.

▸ Surgical consultation is recommended, as there is a risk of abdominal organ incarceration if left unrepaired. A transabdominal surgical approach is now preferred.

Further Reading

Minneci PC, Deans KJ, Kim P, Mathisen DJ. Foramen of Morgagni hernia: changes in diagnosis and treatment. *Ann Thorac Surg.* 2004 Jun;77(6):1956-1959.

History

▶ 37-year-old woman with chest pain and shortness of breath was first imaged with a chest radiograph, which then prompted a chest CT.

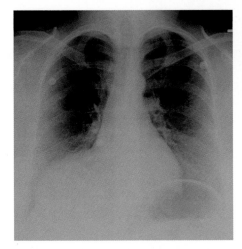

Figure 32.1

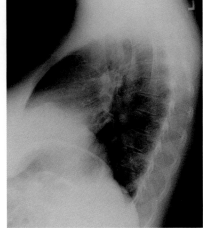

Figure 32.2

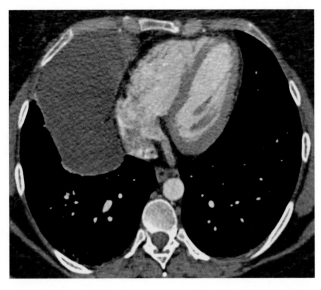

Figure 32.3

Case 32 Pericardial Cyst

Figure 32.4

Figure 32.5

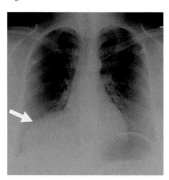 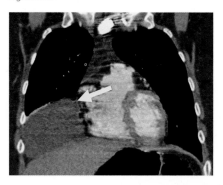

Findings

▶ On the chest radiograph, there is a rounded mass (arrow in Fig. 32.4) centered in the right cardiophrenic angle. The lateral radiograph (Fig. 32.2) confirms that the mass is in the anterior mediastinum.

▶ On the CT (Fig. 32.3), there is a well-circumscribed water-attenuation mass abutting the right heart border and pericardium. Coronal reconstruction provides a nice correlate for the radiograph (Fig. 32.5; arrow denotes the pericardial cyst).

Differential Diagnosis

▶ As with case 31, the differential for a right cardiophrenic angle mass includes pericardial cyst, large pericardial fat pad, adenopathy, mediastinal neoplasm, or foramen of Morgagni hernia.

Teaching Points

▶ Pericardial cysts are one of the most common cardiac masses encountered and most often come to clinical attention incidentally.

▶ Pericardial cysts tend to be homogenous, well-circumscribed, thin-walled, and close to water in attenuation.

▶ They most commonly occur along the right cardiophrenic angle and/or diaphragm.

▶ Communications with the pericardial cavity are usually not seen by routine cross-sectional imaging.

▶ Loculated pericardial effusions can mimic pericardial cysts and occur due to adhesions that have developed in the pericardial space, related to prior surgery or infection. Loculated effusions may change in size over time.

▶ If proteinaceous, the lesion can approach soft tissue in attenuation on CT. MR can be used in these cases to confirm that the lesion is a cyst through heavily T2-weighted sequences (STIR). Gadolinium contrast can be given with subtraction imaging used to exclude internal or wall enhancement.

Management

▶ As these lesions are most often asymptomatic, no further intervention is required. If the lesion becomes symptomatic as a result of mass effect on the heart or adjacent structures, it can be surgically resected.

Further Reading

Wang ZJ, Reddy GP, Gotway MB, et al. CT and MR imaging of pericardial disease. *Radiographics*. 2003 Oct;23 Spec No:S167-180.

History

▸ 33-year-old man presenting with shortness of breath presents to the Emergency Department and receives this radiograph.

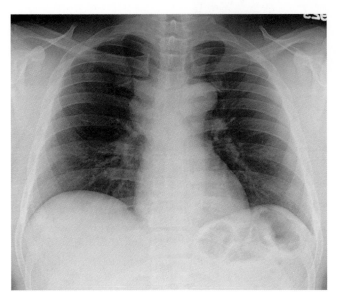

Figure 33.1

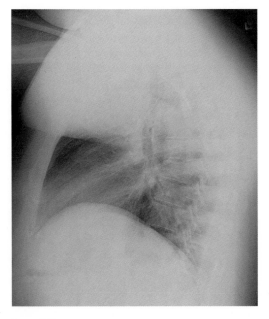

Figure 33.2

Case 33 Intrathoracic Goiter

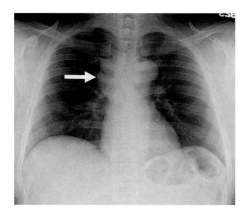

Figure 33.3

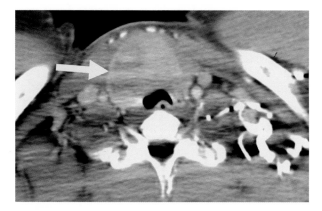

Figure 33.4

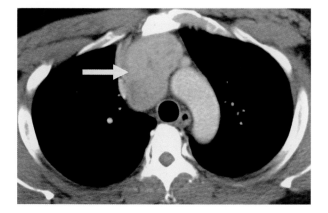

Figure 33.5

Findings

▶ Frontal chest radiograph demonstrates a right paratracheal mass (arrow in Fig. 33.3), which on the lateral view displaces the trachea posteriorly, indicating that the mass lies in either the right paratracheal space or anterior mediastinum. Note that the superior edge of the mass is not well seen.

▶ Subsequent CT demonstrates a heterogeneously enhancing mass (arrows in Figs. 33.4 and 33.5) extending from an enlarged thyroid into the anterior mediastinum. The mass also exerts mass effect on the anterior tracheal wall near the thoracic inlet.

Differential Diagnosis

▶ Based on the chest radiograph, the differential diagnosis would be headed by an anterior mediastinal mass, given that the center of the lesion lies anterior to the trachea. The differential diagnosis would include germ cell tumor and lymphoma, based on the patient's young age. Occasionally, thymoma and goiter may present in younger adults. The CT would be diagnostic of goiter.

Teaching Points

▶ Substernal goiters are common, approaching 15%, depending on how the term "substernal" is defined. There is a low but significant risk of malignancy, ranging from 3% to 21%.

▶ While often symptomatic, large goiters can present with airway compromise or due to vascular compression.

▶ Approximately 1% of goiters are considered primary retrosternal lesions with no communication with the cervical thyroid. Secondary retrosternal goiters that communicate with the cervical thyroid may display a cervicothoracic sign (extension of the mass above the thoracic inlet) in which the superior margin is ill defined due to blending with neck soft tissues, unlike the case of a posterior mediastinal mass, which is nicely outlined by the apical portions of the lung.

Management

▶ Surgical resection is the treatment of choice. In experienced hands, almost all lesions can be resected via a cervical approach, avoiding median sternotomy.

Further Reading

Cohen JP. Substernal goiters and sternotomy. *Laryngoscope*. 2009;119:683-688.

History

▶ 40-year-old man with recently diagnosed head and neck squamous cell carcinoma undergoes CT for preoperative staging.

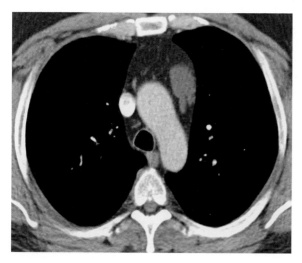

Figure 34.1

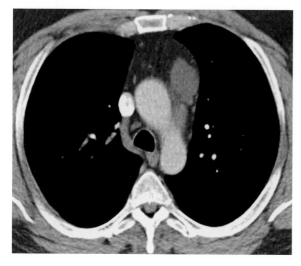

Figure 34.2

Case 34 Thymic Cyst

Figure 34.3

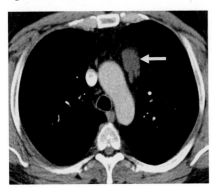

Figure 34.4

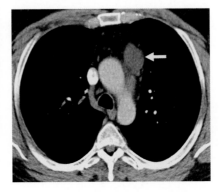

Findings

▶ CT uncovered a well-defined, lobulated, homogeneous, fluid-attenuation lesion (arrows in Figs. 34.3 and 34.4) centered in the anterior mediastinum.

Differential Diagnosis

▶ Based on the location and fluid attenuation, the differential diagnosis includes thymic cyst, pericardial cyst, and loculated fluid in a pericardial recess. Given the clear separation from the pericardium, thymic cyst would be favored.

Teaching Points

▶ The majority of thymic cysts are incidentally detected lesions thought to arise congenitally from embryonic remnants along the thymopharyngeal duct from the upper neck to the anterior mediastinum.

▶ Thymic cysts may also occur in the setting of mediastinal radiation or chemotherapy.

▶ Thymic cysts should be fluid in attenuation, but occasionally they will be higher in attenuation due to hemorrhage or proteinaceous debris. If soft tissue nodularity is present, cystic neoplasms must be considered, such as teratoma, cystic thymoma, or necrotic lymphoma.

▶ Occasionally multiple cysts may be seen in the thymus. These lymphoepithelial cysts may be seen in HIV/AIDS or as a manifestation of Langerhans cell histiocytosis (especially in children).

Management

▶ Thymic cysts require no intervention, as they are most commonly incidentally detected.

Further Reading

Nasseri F, Eftekhari F. Clinical and radiologic review of the normal and abnormal thymus: pearls and pitfalls. *Radiographics*. 2010;30: 413-428.

History

▶ 35-year-old with chest pain and shortness of breath.

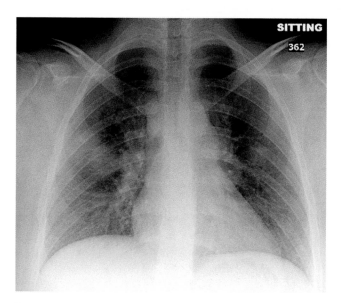

Figure 35.1

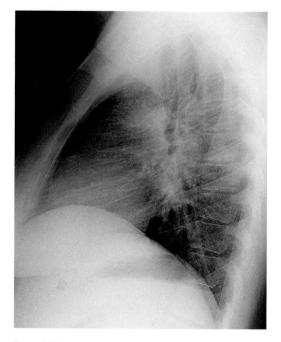

Figure 35.2

Case 35 Mediastinal Lymphadenopathy (Sarcoidosis)

Figure 35.3

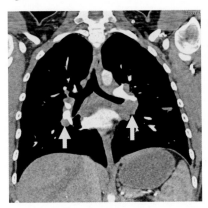

Figure 35.4

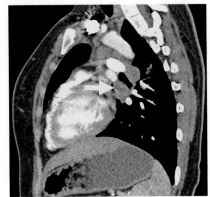

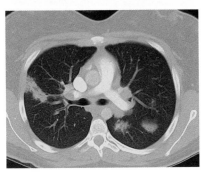

Figure 35.5

Findings

▶ The frontal radiograph demonstrates bilateral lobulated hila in keeping with hilar lymphadenopathy. Right paratracheal lymphadenopathy and aorticopulmonary lymphadenopathy are also seen.
▶ The lateral radiograph demonstrates a circular opacity surrounding the mainstem bronchi (*doughnut sign*). This ring is in keeping with middle mediastinal lymphadenopathy.
▶ CT confirms the lymphadenopathy (arrows in Figs. 35.3 and 35.4). Parenchymal opacities are also seen on the lung windows (Fig. 35.5).

Differential Diagnosis

▶ Mediastinal lymphadenopathy can be seen in the setting of granulomatous infection, granulomatous inflammation (sarcoid), or neoplasm (lymphoma or metastases). The homogenous attenuation, lack of vascular occlusion, symmetry in the mediastinum, parenchymal opacities, and young age would favor sarcoidosis.

Teaching Points

▶ On a chest radiograph, the right paratracheal stripe should be <4 mm. When larger, a mediastinal mass (usually lymphadenopathy) should be suspected.
▶ The aorticopulmonary window (the left mediastinal border between the aorta and main pulmonary artery) should be concave. When it is convex, a mediastinal mass (usually lymphadenopathy) should be suspected.
▶ Distinguishing enlarged pulmonary arteries from hilar lymphadenopathy can be challenging. The visualization of an inferior border is a useful finding in lymphadenopathy; it is not seen with enlarged vessels.

- Lymphadenopathy may be easily missed on the frontal examination, but using the lateral examination to look for the doughnut sign can be helpful.
- CT is useful in determining the location and pattern of the lymphadenopathy and lung findings that will direct the differential diagnosis. Calcification, enhancement, and low attenuation are features that can help refine the differential diagnosis on CT.
- Sarcoidosis tends to involve the right paratracheal and bilateral lymph nodes. This is sometimes referred to as a one-two-three pattern.
- Lymphadenopathy in sarcoidosis tends to be homogeneous and soft tissue in attenuation without compression of adjacent vasculature or bronchi.

Management

- Further evaluation in this situation would begin with transbronchial biopsy. Right paratracheal nodes can be sampled by conventional mediastinoscopy. Increasingly, endoscopic bronchoscopic ultrasound (EBUS) is being used for hilar node sampling.

Further Reading

Sharma A, Fidias P, Hayman LA, et al. Patterns of lymphadenopathy in thoracic malignancies. *Radiographics*. 2004 Mar-Apr; 24(2): 419-434.

History

▶ 43-year-old woman is admitted with chest pain.

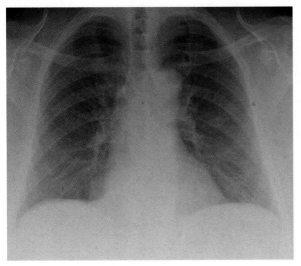

Figure 36.1

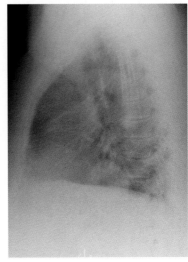

Figure 36.2

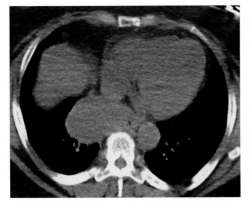

Figure 36.3

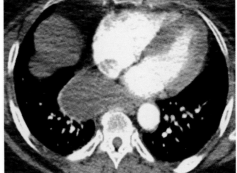

Figure 36.4

Case 36 Esophageal Duplication Cyst

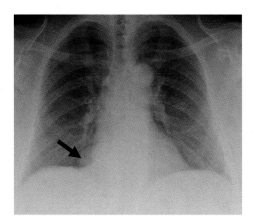

Figure 36.5

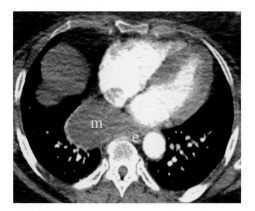

Figure 36.6

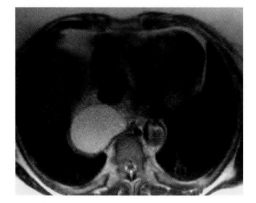

Figure 36.7

Findings

▶ The chest radiograph demonstrates a well-circumscribed mass in the right costophrenic angle (arrow in Fig. 36.5). On the lateral view, the mass projects over the middle mediastinum (Fig. 36.2).

▶ CT demonstrates a well-circumscribed mass in the middle mediastinum that does not enhance and is uniformly low in attenuation. The mass (m) abuts the esophagus (e) in Figure 36.6.

▶ T2-weighted MRI (Fig. 36.7) demonstrates increased uniform fluid intensity within the mass, which is similar to cerebrospinal fluid. There is no associated soft tissue component.

Differential Diagnosis

▶ The differential diagnosis for a middle mediastinal mass includes a foregut duplication cyst, esophageal mass, lymphadenopathy, or a vascular lesion. The CT appearance with uniform low attenuation and no enhancement is characteristic of a duplication cyst.

Teaching Points

▶ Often it may be difficult to differentiate bronchogenic cyst from esophageal duplication cyst on imaging. For this reason, some favor the use of a more generic term, *foregut duplication cyst*.

▶ A bronchogenic cyst will contain respiratory epithelium and cartilage, whereas an esophageal duplication cyst will be lined with smooth muscle and will not contain cartilage. An infected or hemorrhagic cyst will result in denuded and featureless epithelium.

▶ 50% or more of esophageal duplication cysts have attenuation greater than water from protein or blood products.

▶ If CT demonstrates a well-circumscribed mass that has a thin wall and measures fluid attenuation (<15 HU), no further imaging evaluation is required.

▶ MR is useful in complex duplication cysts because uniform high signal will be seen on the T2 sequence. The T1 signal will be variable due to the content of protein and blood products.

▶ Most bronchogenic cysts are found in the subcarinal or right paratracheal regions. Esophageal duplication cysts can occur anywhere along the course of the esophagus.

Management

▶ As duplication cysts can increase in size from infection or hemorrhage, they are often resected. Some surgeons have also advocated aspiration for treatment and diagnosis; however, the cysts may recur following aspiration.

Further Reading

McAdams HP, Kirejczyk WM, Rosado-de-Christenson ML, et al. Bronchogenic cyst: imaging features with clinical and histopathologic correlation. *Radiology*. Nov. 2000;217(2):441-446.

History

▶ 49-year-old woman presents with shoulder pain.

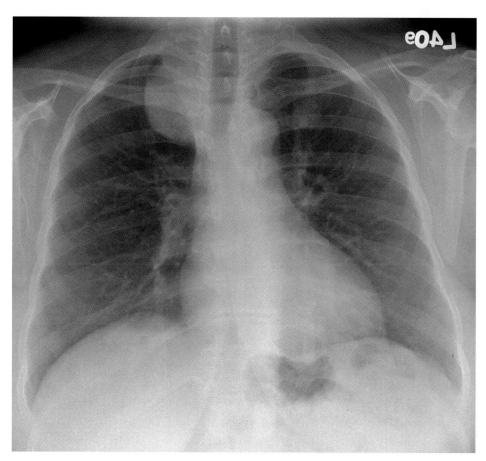

Figure 37.1

Case 37   Posterior Mediastinal Mass (Schwannoma)

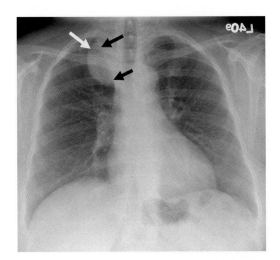

Figure 37.2

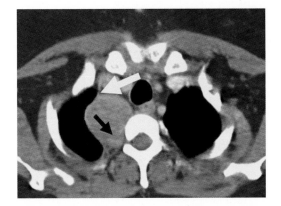

Figure 37.3

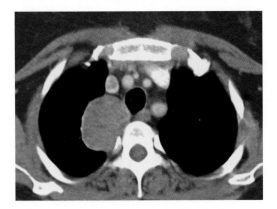

Figure 37.4

Findings

▶ The radiograph demonstrates a right paratracheal mass extending above the clavicle (white arrow in Fig. 37.2). Splaying of the posterior right fourth and fifth ribs is also seen.

▶ Black arrows in Figure 37.2 show the interface of the mass with the lung (mediastinal border), which creates an obtuse angle, suggesting a mediastinal lesion.

▶ CT (Figs. 37.3 and 37.4) confirms the mass to be posterior mediastinal. The mass subtly enhances (black arrow in Fig. 37.3). White arrow in Figure 37.3 shows that the interface with the lung creates an obtuse angle.

Differential Diagnosis

▶ Differential diagnosis is based on a posterior mediastinal mass. In an adult, a nerve sheath tumor would lead the differential diagnosis. Other causes of posterior mediastinal masses, including extramedullary hematopoiesis, lateral meningocele, and vertebral osteomyelitis/diskitis are not likely.

Teaching Points

▶ The *cervicothoracic sign* refers to the superior extension of the mass above the clavicles. Because the anterior lung stops at the level of the clavicles, a mass demonstrating this sign must be posterior in the thorax or arising from the neck.

▶ Posterior mediastinal lesions are considered to be neurogenic until proven otherwise. In an adult, they tend to be of nerve sheath origin (neurofibroma, schwannoma, or neurolemmoma). In children and young adults, they may be of sympathetic ganglia origin (ganglioneuroma, neuroblastoma, ganglioneuroblastoma).

▶ Nerve sheath tumors tend to be one or two rib interspaces in z-axis, while sympathetic ganglia tumors are longer.

▶ Schwannomas and neurofibromas are well circumscribed and round. Because of myelin and occasional cystic regions, they tend to be lower than muscle in CT attenuation. On MR, they tend to be higher than muscle on T2 and often enhance with a targetoid appearance.

▶ Neural foraminal enlargement may not be seen with nerve sheath tumors, but osseous remodeling is common.

▶ Schwannomas are usually incidental, but one third of patients with neurofibromas will have neurofibromatosis.

Management

▶ These may be resected because of local symptoms. The risk of malignant transformation is low in isolated schwannomas.

Further Reading

Whitten C, Khan S, Munneke G, et al. Diagnostic approach to mediastinal abnormalities. *Radiographics.* 2007;27:657-671.

History

► 56-year-old man presents with pleuritic chest pain and back pain.

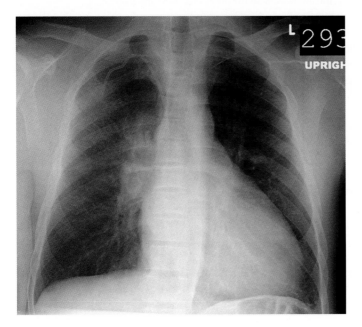

Figure 38.1

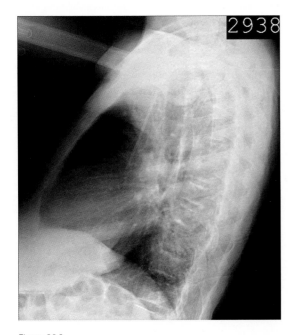

Figure 38.2

Case 38 Discitis

Figure 38.3

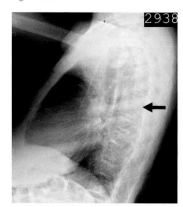

Figure 38.4

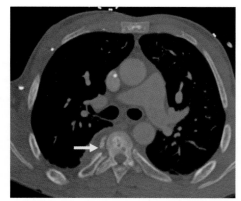

Figure 38.5

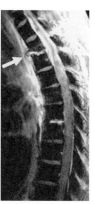

Findings

▸ Chest radiograph shows right hilar density, which is centered over the midthoracic spine on the lateral. Loss of disc space height and endplate destruction of the midthoracic spine (arrow in Fig. 38.3) are also seen.

▸ CT demonstrates the paraspinal soft tissue mass and fluid (arrow in Fig. 38.4) consistent with a phlegmon and developing abscess. MR demonstrates enhancement of the disc space (arrow in Fig. 38.5) with associated abscess.

Differential Diagnosis

▸ Posterior mediastinal masses are usually neurogenic, but also include osteomyelitis of the vertebra, discitis, and extramedullary hematopoiesis. The destruction of the disc space and the soft tissue findings would be supportive of discitis/osteomyelitis.

Teaching Points

▸ Discitis/osteomyelitis of the thoracic spine is an uncommon cause of chest and back pain. It represents one of the more common missed findings in patients receiving CT for chest pain evaluation in the emergency department.

▸ Discitis may have an indolent course and may not present with fever and chills.

▸ It often arises from the hematogenous spread of infection from another site, usually *Staphylococcus aureus.*

▸ Infection tends to begin in the disc space and may spread to involve the adjacent vertebra. Left untreated, the infection will lead to vertebral collapse.

▸ CT findings are better appreciated on sagittal and coronal reconstructions and include endplate destruction and adjacent soft tissue phlegmon or stranding.

▸ MR is better than CT for diagnosing early disease. MR findings include increased T2 signal in the disc and adjacent vertebra with enhancement after the use of gadolinium.

▸ Involvement of one level associated with endplate loss (in addition to remodeling) can be helpful in distinguishing discitis from degenerative disc disease.

▸ Discitis from atypical organisms (including mycobacterial infection) may involve more than one level.

Management

▸ The diagnosis of discitis should be confirmed with biopsy and culture, which can be done under imaging guidance. The cultures are useful to guide antibiotic therapy.

▸ In more advanced cases, surgical débridement and stabilization may be required.

Further Reading

Hillen TJ, Wessell DE. Multidetector CT scan in the evaluation of chest pain of nontraumatic musculoskeletal origin. *Radiol Clin North Am.* 2010 Jan;48(1):185-191.

History

▶ 40-year-old woman with sickle cell disease presents with chest pain.

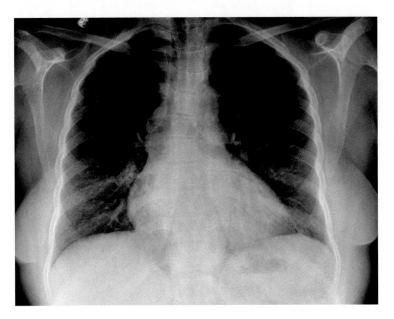

Figure 39.1

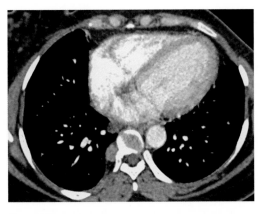

Figure 39.2

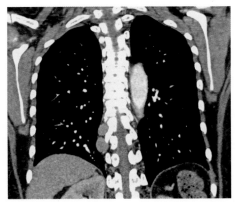

Figure 39.3

Case 39   Extramedullary Hematopoiesis

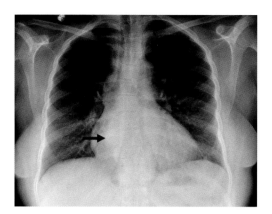

Figure 39.4

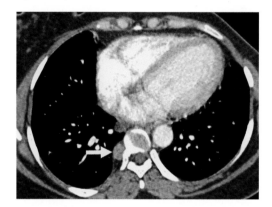

Figure 39.5

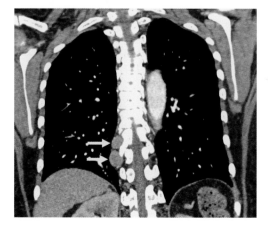

Figure 39.6

Findings

▶ Chest radiograph (Fig. 39.4) demonstrates a right paraspinal soft tissue density that extends three vertebral body levels (arrow). There is no associated rib notching or widening.

▶ Subsequent CT confirms right paravertebral soft tissue masses (arrows in Figs. 39.5 and 39.6) without adjacent bone destruction. No calcium or fat attenuation is seen within the masses.

Differential Diagnosis

▶ The main differential diagnosis for a posterior mediastinal mass includes neurogenic tumor (nerve sheath tumor in adults), lymphadenopathy, and extramedullary hematopoiesis (EMH). Discitis and osseous metastasis are not within the differential list because of an absence of bone findings. Given the history of anemia in sickle cell disease, EMH would be favored.

Teaching Points

▶ EMH is due to red blood cell destruction or lack of production and can be seen in spherocytosis, thalassemia, or other congenital anemias. It is rarely seen with sickle cell disease, myelofibrosis, or leukemias/lymphomas.

▶ EMH usually results in bilateral paravertebral masses that do not connect. The lack of a connection or isthmus suggests that the masses arose independently and that a lesion did not simply grow to the other side.

▶ The diagnosis of EMH can be confirmed with a Tc-99m sulfur colloid study, which will demonstrate uptake in bone marrow-producing elements.

▶ Marrow expansion, which can be seen with EMH, may result in coarsened bone trabeculation, especially in the vertebrae and ribs.

▶ EMH may be seen almost anywhere, including the liver, spleen, peritoneum, pleura, and bladder.

▶ When the anemia resolves, the areas of EMH may take on fat attenuation.

Management

▶ Once the diagnosis is established, no treatment is required, other than for supportive care for the patient's anemia.

▶ In the rare circumstance that the hematopoiesis is resulting in local mass effect, decompressive treatment would be needed.

Further Reading

Gogia P, Goel R, Nayar S. Extramedullary paraspinal hematopoiesis in hereditary spherocytsosis. *Ann Thorac Med.* 2008;3(2):64-66.
Lall C, Payne DK. A patient with anemia and a paraspinal chest mass. *Chest.* 2003;124(2):732-734.

History

▶ 30-year-old woman with a history of bone marrow transplant for lymphoma presents with chest pain.

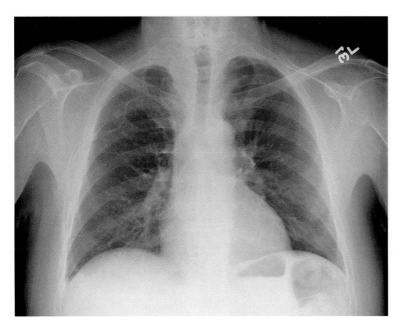

Figure 40.1

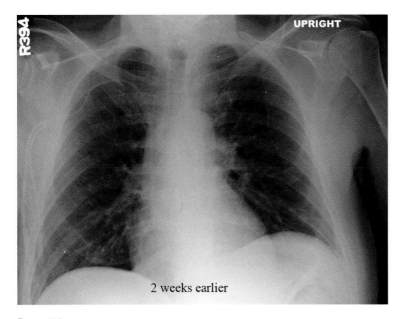

Figure 40.2

Case 40 Acute Mediastinitis

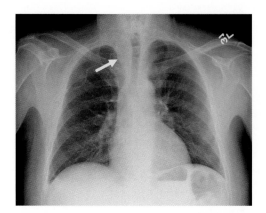

Figure 40.3

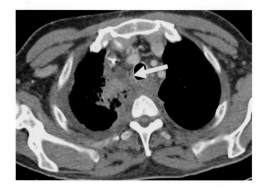

Figure 40.4

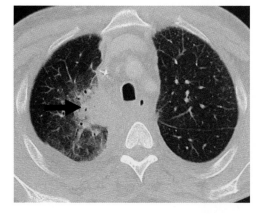

Figure 40.5

Findings

▸ The chest radiograph demonstrates a right paratracheal soft tissue density with mass effect on the trachea (white arrow in Fig. 40.3). This mass has developed in a 2-week interval.

▸ CT images demonstrate a right upper lobe consolidation (arrow in Fig. 40.4). There is loss of the normal fat planes within the mediastinum accompanied by an increase in attenuation of the mediastinal fat at the level of the consolidation (arrow in Fig. 40.5).

Differential Diagnosis

▸ Rapid increase in mediastinal size can be seen in the setting of hematoma and mediastinitis. The clinical history can be very helpful in making the distinction. The absence of trauma and recent line placement would favor the latter. Rarely, aggressive leukemia or lymphoma can present with change in the mediastinal size in less than 1 month.

Teaching Points

▸ Acute mediastinitis usually results from perforation of the esophagus or cardiac surgery, but may also result from extension of pneumonia, retropharyngeal infection, or sternoclavicular septic arthritis.

▸ Acute necrotizing mediastinitis has a very high mortality, with reported rates of 30% to 50%.

▸ CT is helpful in evaluating the presence of fluid collections that may need to be drained.

▸ Occasionally on CT pneumomediastinum may be seen. Mediastinal fat stranding and enlargement are almost always present.

▸ The postoperative mediastinum can be very difficult to distinguish from acute mediastinitis. Fluid and gas collections in the noninfected, postoperative mediastinum, however, should begin to resolve by 3 weeks.

▸ Particular attention needs to be paid for the evaluation of an esophageal perforation, as this requires urgent surgical intervention and carries a high mortality even if treated.

Management

▸ Treatment is based on correcting the underlying etiology (perforated esophagus, septic arthritis, cellulitis) but may also consist of percutaneous drainage if any abscesses are present. Antibiotics are always instituted.

Further Reading

Athanassiadi KA. Infections of the mediastinum. *Thorac Surg Clin.* 2009 Feb;19(1):37-45.

Exarhos DN, Malagari K, Tsatalou EG, et al. Acute mediastinitis: spectrum of computed tomography findings. *Eur Radiol.* 2005 Aug;15(8):1569-1574.

History

▶ 31-year-old man presents with progressive shortness of breath.

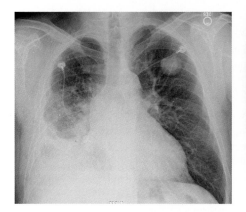

Figure 41.1

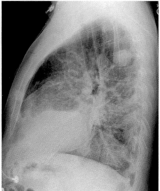

Figure 41.2

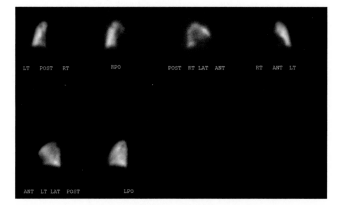

Figure 41.3

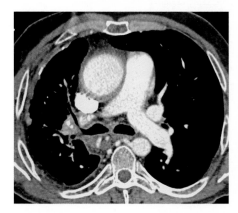

Figure 41.4

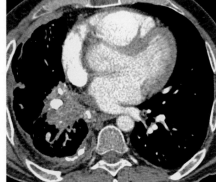

Figure 41.5

Case 41　Fibrosing Mediastinitis

Figure 41.6

Figure 41.7

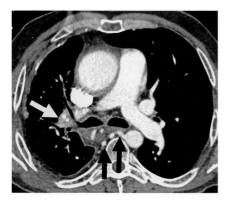

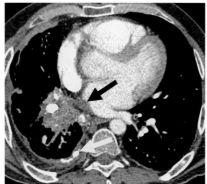

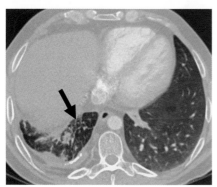

Figure 41.8

Findings

▶ Chest radiograph (Figs. 41.1 and 41.2) demonstrates right volume loss with associated lymphadenopathy, pleural thickening, and unilateral interstitial edema. Perfusion images (Fig. 41.3) show absent right perfusion.

▶ CT shows an infiltrative right hilar process with some associated calcification (white arrow in Fig. 41.6; black arrow in Fig. 41.7). The mass obliterates the right pulmonary arteries and veins. (Black arrow in Fig. 41.7 denotes the location in which the right inferior pulmonary vein should be seen.) Associated calcified pleural thickening is seen (white arrow in Fig. 41.7).

▶ Right bronchial arteries are enlarged (black arrows in Fig. 41.6) and right septal line thickening is seen (black arrow in Fig. 41.8).

Differential Diagnosis

▶ The main differential consists of fibrosing mediastinitis (FM), lung cancer (most notably small cell cancer), and lymphoma. The presence of a large granuloma, calcified pleural plaques, and calcification favors FM.

Teaching Points

▶ FM refers to idiopathic dense fibrous tissue within the mediastinum.

▶ In the United States, most cases are associated with histoplasmosis infection. The histoplasmosis antigen incites an autoimmune fibrotic reaction.

▶ Other associations include infections (fungal or mycobacterial), autoimmune diseases, and medications.

▶ Patients present with compressive symptoms on the superior vena cava, pulmonary veins, or pulmonary arteries.

- The bronchi are usually affected after the veins and arteries.
- FM tends to be unilateral (usually the right side) and may result in unilateral absence of perfusion.
- Bronchial collaterals are usually seen and may result in hemoptysis as a presenting symptom.
- Rarely, FM can compress the coronary arteries, resulting in coronary ischemia, or the esophagus, creating symptoms of dysphagia.
- On CT, calcification is often present but not required. In the more diffuse form of FM (which is not as clearly associated with prior infection), calcification is less common.

Management

- When the radiographic appearance is characteristic, no biopsy may be performed. Biopsy may be performed to exclude neoplasm. Rarely are organisms retrieved.
- Management is directed at relieving the vascular compromise. This includes stenting and angioplasty.

Further Reading

Rossi SE, McAdams HP, Rosado-de-Christenson ML, et al. Fibrosing mediastinitis. *Radiographics*. 2001;21:737-757.

History

▶ 12-year-old boy presents with malaise and fevers.

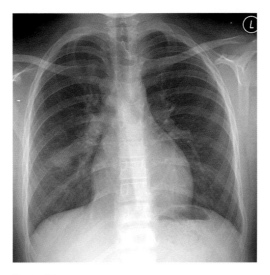

Figure 42.1

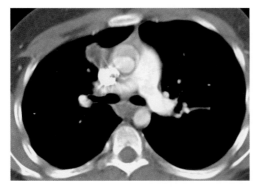

Figure 42.2

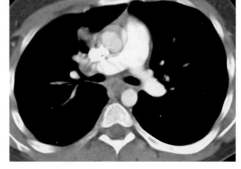

Figure 42.3

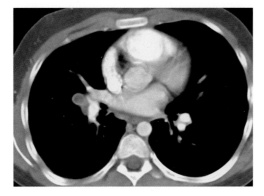

Figure 42.4

Case 42   Low-attenuation Lymph Nodes (Histoplasmosis)

Figure 42.5

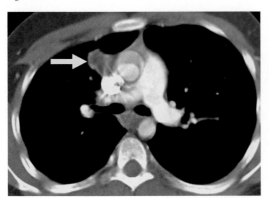

Figure 42.6

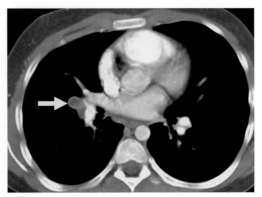

Findings

▶ Original frontal radiograph (Fig. 42.1) shows mediastinal lymphadenopathy and patchy right middle lobe atelectasis.
▶ Subsequent CT with intravenous contrast confirmed the lymphadenopathy but also showed low-attenuating centers within the mediastinal nodes (arrows in Figs. 42.5 and 42.6) and rim enhancement.

Differential Diagnosis

▶ The differential diagnosis for low-attenuating lymphadenopathy includes infectious granulomatous disease (tuberculosis or histoplasmosis), but also includes lymphoma and metastases. In a previously healthy young patient with no history of cancer, granulomatous infection would be favored.

Teaching Points

▶ Low-attenuating lymph nodes are defined as lymph nodes with lower attenuation than the skeletal muscle seen on the same image.
▶ A thin rind of peripheral enhancement with a low-attenuating, necrotic center is suggestive of active granulomatous inflammation (either histoplasmosis or tuberculosis).
▶ Lymph nodal involvement by mycobacterial or fungal disease may occur without pulmonary involvement. This is especially true in children.
▶ In HIV-positive patients, sometimes *Mycobacterium avium intracellulare* can present with low-attenuating, rim-enhancing lymphadenopathy.
▶ Occasionally lymphoma and metastases (lung, seminoma, gastric, or ovarian) can present with low-attenuating lymphadenopathy. About 25% of lymphomas will present this way.
▶ Rarely, Whipple's disease will present with low-attenuating lymph nodes, which are closer to fat in attenuation. This infectious arthropathy is associated with small bowel findings and has fat-containing nodes from an abundance of macrophages.
▶ Another unusual mimic is plexiform neurofibromas in the setting of neurofibromatosis. These nerve sheath tumors are myelin-rich and are, therefore, low in attenuation on CT.

Management

▶ The possibility of acute tuberculosis requires the patient to be placed in isolation until proven not contagious. A PPD should be placed and the sputum collected for culture and microscopic evaluation.
▶ Patients may undergo bronchoscopy and biopsy for culture, if the diagnosis cannot be made less invasively. In this case, transbronchial biopsy was required to make the diagnosis.

Further Reading

Suwatanapongched T, Gierada D. CT of thoracic lymph nodes. Part II: diseases and pitfalls. *Br J Radiol.* 2006;79:999-1000.

History

▶ 49-year-old man with weight loss is imaged to find a potential etiology.

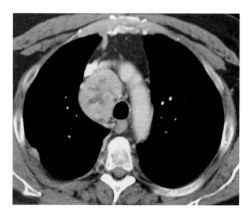

Figure 43.1

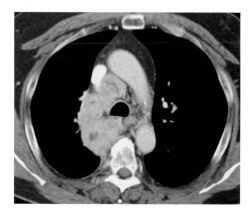

Figure 43.2

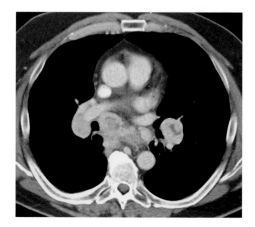

Figure 43.3

Case 43 Hyperenhancing Lymphadenopathy (from Metastatic Renal Cell Carcinoma)

Figure 43.4

Figure 43.5

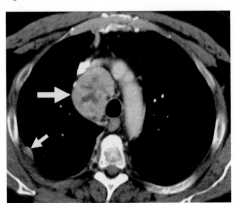
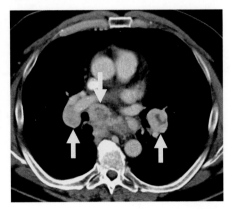

Findings

▶ Right paratracheal, bilateral hilar and subcarinal enhancing adenopathy (white arrows in Figs. 43.4 and 43.5) is seen. A pleural deposit is also noted in the right upper hemothorax (smaller arrow in Fig. 43.4).

▶ Images of the upper abdomen (not shown) revealed changes of right nephrectomy.

Differential Diagnosis

▶ Hypervascular lymphadenopathy is defined as lymph nodes that enhance more than skeletal muscle. It can be seen in hypervascular metastases (especially renal cell carcinoma, melanoma, and thyroid cancers) and Castleman disease (CD).

Teaching Points

▶ Highly vascular metastases should be high on the differential diagnosis of enhancing lymph nodes.

▶ CD, or angiofollicular lymph node hyperplasia, falls in the spectrum of lymph node hyperplasias of uncertain etiology. It can be divided into hyaline vascular types and plasma cell types.

▶ Hyaline vascular CD most commonly presents as unicentric disease with a dominant, often mediastinal, nodal mass or conglomerate without systemic symptoms and is the most common form.

▶ Plasma cell CD commonly presents with multicentric disease, involving multiple nodal stations in the neck, chest, and/or abdomen, along with systemic symptoms of fever, weight loss, and anemia. Patients with Kaposi sarcoma and HIV have a higher incidence of CD.

▶ Multicentric CD can progress to lymphoma or can predispose to infectious complications, given the heightened inflammatory response.

Management

▶ Evaluation for known hypervascular primary malignancies is necessary, possibly requiring whole body CT or PET-CT.

▶ If CD is considered in the differential diagnosis, surgical excision is usually necessary as the architectural details of the node required for diagnosis cannot be obtained with fine-needle aspiration. Surgical excision is usually curative in unicentric hyaline vascular CD, whereas multicentric plasma cell CD is treated with a combination of chemotherapy, immunosuppression/steroids, and/or radiation.

Further Reading

McAdams HP, Rosado-de-Christenson M, Fishback NF, Templeton PA. Castleman disease of the thorax: radiologic features with clinical and histopathologic correlation. *Radiology*. 1998 Oct;209(1):221-228.

History

▶ 22-year-old man complains of intractable nausea and vomiting.

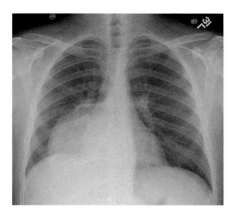

Figure 44.1

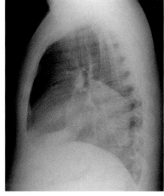

Figure 44.2

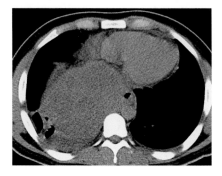

Figure 44.3

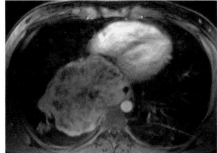

Figure 44.4

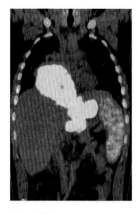

Figure 44.5

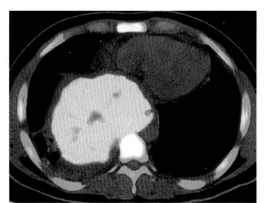

Figure 44.6

113

Case 44 Mediastinal Myofibroblastic Tumor

Findings

▶ The admission chest radiograph shows a mass eccentrically situated in the middle mediastinum (Figs. 44.1 and 44.2). This is not a cardiophrenic angle mass, because it sits posterior to the heart.
▶ The chest CT (Fig. 44.3) was performed without intravenous contrast but was followed by a contrast-enhanced MR (Fig. 44.4). These studies both show that the mass is eccentrically situated compared to the esophagus and associated with a small pleural effusion.
▶ The MR shows heterogeneous contrast enhancement.
▶ The lesion is markedly FDG-avid on the PET images (Figs. 44.5 and 44.6).

Differential Diagnosis

▶ The differential diagnosis of a middle mediastinal lesion includes lymphadenopathy, vascular anomaly, and duplication cyst. Given the large size, FDG avidity, and contrast enhancement, malignancy such as spindle cell neoplasm should also be considered (and favored).

Teaching Points

▶ When a middle mediastinal lesion becomes large and enhances heterogeneously, the differential diagnosis must include spindle cell neoplasms. More commonly, these may be stromal tumors of the esophagus (leiomyomas, leiomyosarcomas, or gastrointestinal stromal tumors). In a patient of this age, an inflammatory myofibroblastic tumor (formerly known as pseudotumor) should also be considered. If the lesion contains fat, one should consider liposarcoma. A history of neurofibromatosis may prompt the consideration of a neurofibroma/sarcoma.
▶ Spindle cell neoplasms of the mediastinum can involve any compartment (anterior, middle, or posterior), although the middle mediastinum tends to be the most common site.
▶ Inflammatory myofibroblastic tumor (IMT) represents one type of inflammatory pseudotumor that is believed to be from a proliferation of myofibroblasts. In other words, it is not a pseudotumor but a true tumor. The myofibroblasts are usually seen against a background of inflammatory cells.
▶ The IMT represents the most common primary lung neoplasm in children.
▶ IMT may arise in any part of the body. The symptoms will be based on the affected organs.
▶ Local invasion is rare but has been reported, and occasionally the IMT may metastasize. Growing literature suggests that these more aggressive IMTs may be associated with chromosomal mutations.
▶ IMTs are best thought of as neoplasms of borderline malignant potential with a rare possibility of aggressive behavior.

Management

▶ Local resection is the only cure. Spontaneous regression has been reported, but these tumors tend not be responsive to chemotherapy or radiation.

Further Reading

Dehner LP. The enigmatic inflammatory pseudotumours: the current state of our understanding, or misunderstanding. *J Pathol.* 2000 Nov;192(3):277-279.

History

▶ 71-year-old man with cough and abnormal chest radiograph is referred for CT.

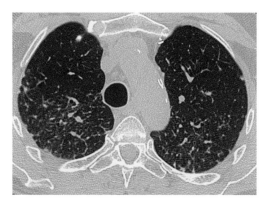

Figure 45.1

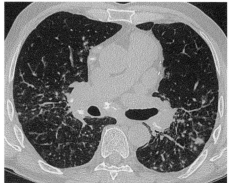

Figure 45.2

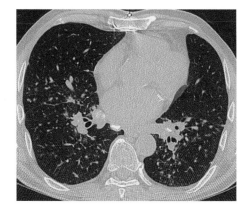

Figure 45.3

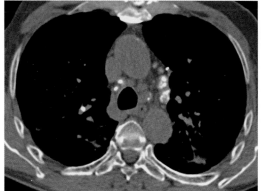

Figure 45.4

Case 45 Silicosis (with Eggshell Calcifications in Mediastinal Lymph Nodes)

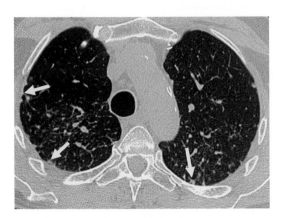

Figure 45.5

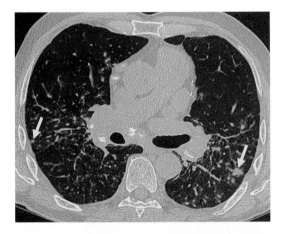

Figure 45.6

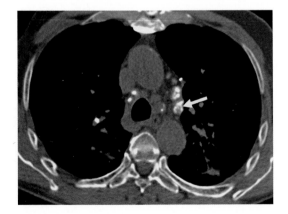

Figure 45.7

Findings

▶ Perilymphatic micronodules (arrows in Figs. 45.5 and 45.6), some of which touch the pleural surface, are seen in a middle and upper lung distribution. Peripherally calcified (egg-shell calcified) mediastinal lymph nodes (arrow in Fig. 45.7) are also seen.

Differential Diagnosis

▶ Eggshell calcifications can be seen in sarcoidosis, silicosis, prior tuberculosis, or treated lymphomas. Given the perilymphatic nodules, silicosis (especially in a patient of this age) and sarcoidosis would be favored.

Teaching Points

▶ Micronodules touching the pleura can be seen in perilymphatic diseases (silicosis, sarcoidosis, or lymphangitic tumor spread) and miliary disease (metastases, infectious granulomatous disease); however, perilymphatic nodules are clustered in the lung as opposed to the uniformly distributed nodules seen in miliary disease.

▶ Silicosis results from exposure to silica particles, commonly seen in mining, tunneling, rock cutting, and sandblasting professions. Generally, findings are not present until 10 or 15 years after exposure.

▶ Silica is deposited in alveoli, where it is taken up by macrophages, which subsequently die and elicit a fibrotic response. Simple, uncomplicated silicosis manifests as small (1–2 mm) micronodules in a perilymphatic distribution in the upper peripheral lungs. Over time, these nodules may coalesce along the pleural surface, leading to pseudo-plaques.

▶ In complicated silicosis, parenchymal nodules can coalesce into large (1 cm or greater) opacities (progressive massive fibrosis) that retract over time towards the hila.

▶ When lymph nodes calcify with a thin peripheral rim, the pattern is often referred to as *eggshell calcification*. Lymph nodes with eggshell calcifications can be seen in sarcoidosis, silicosis, treated lymphomas (most notably Hodgkin's disease), and tuberculosis.

Management

▶ Exposure history is important in the establishment of occupational lung diseases. Transbronchial biopsy may be performed to exclude the diagnosis of sarcoidosis, which is usually the main alternative.

Further Reading

Kim KI, Kim CW, Lee MK, et al. Imaging of occupational lung disease. *Radiographics*. 2001 Nov-Dec;21(6):1371-1391.

Sirajuddin A, Kanne JP. Occupational lung disease. *J Thorac Imaging*. 2009 Nov;24(4):310-320.

Part 4   Tracheal Cases

History

▶ 60-year-old man with history of chewing tobacco for 34 years and 3 pack-year smoking presents with stridor and cough.

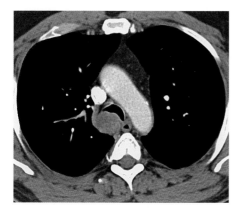

Figure 46.1

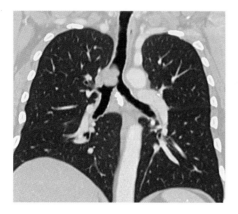

Figure 46.2

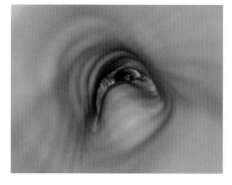

Figure 46.3

Case 46 Tracheal Tumor (Adenoid Cystic Carcinoma)

Findings

▶ CT shows a mass arising from the posterolateral wall of the trachea, causing marked luminal narrowing (Fig. 46.1). The mass invades the tracheal wall and extends into the mediastinum. The mass is homogeneous without calcification.

▶ Multiplanar reformatting is useful in displaying the craniocaudal extent of the lesion and the relationship of the mass with the carina (Fig. 46.2). This mass involves a short segment of the trachea and extends into the right mainstem bronchus.

▶ Volume rendering provides a "virtual bronchoscopic" view of the lesion (Fig. 46.3).

Differential Diagnosis

▶ Invasion of the tracheal wall with extension into the mediastinum should lead one to suspect a malignant neoplasm: squamous cell carcinoma or adenoid cystic carcinoma (ACC). Other considerations include local invasion by adjacent tumor, such as thyroid, lung, or esophageal cancer, and hematogenous metastases, most commonly sarcoma, melanoma, renal, breast, and hematologic malignancies, such as leukemia.

Teaching Points

▶ ACC of the trachea arises from the minor salivary glands, located in the posterolateral aspect of the tracheal wall.

▶ ACC is the second most common malignant neoplasm of the trachea after squamous cell carcinoma.

▶ Unlike squamous cell carcinoma, ACC has no association with smoking.

▶ ACC commonly grows along the perineural and submucosal planes, such that it can cause circumferential and long segment tracheal wall thickening. Because of this growth pattern, it was formerly referred to as a cylindroma.

▶ ACC has a better prognosis than squamous cell carcinoma because it grows slowly and regional lymphadenopathy and distant metastases are rare.

▶ If distant metastases occur, they present late in the course of disease.

Management

▶ Surgical resection is performed when there is no distant metastasis or when the tumor involves six or fewer tracheal rings, allowing successful subsequent anastomosis. Chemotherapy, radiation, and palliative measures may be used to maintain airway patency when surgical resection cannot be done.

Further Reading

Javidan-Nejad C. MDCT of trachea and main bronchi. *Radiol Clin North Am.* 2010 Jan;48(1):157-176.

Spizarny DL, Shepard JA, McLoud TC, et al. CT of adenoid cystic carcinoma of the trachea. *AJR Am J Roentgenol.* 1986 Jun;146(6): 1129-1132.

History

▶ 75-year-old woman with refractory cough presents for CT.

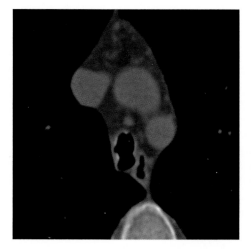

Figure 47.1

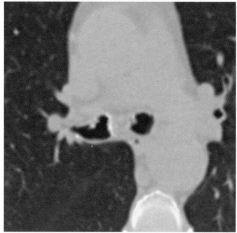

Figure 47.2

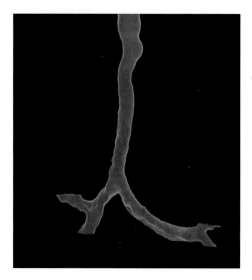

Figure 47.3

Case 47   Tracheobronchopathia Osteochondroplastica (TPOP)

Findings

▶ Non contrast CT images of the trachea and main bronchi demonstrate hyperattenuating nodules protruding into the airway lumen. Note that the posterior membrane of the trachea is spared in Figure 47.1.

▶ The irregularity of the tracheal wall and long segment involvement of trachea and both mainstem bronchi are shown with the volume-rendered image (Fig. 47.3).

Differential Diagnosis

▶ Causes of nodular and diffuse luminal narrowing include TPOP, amyloidosis, papillomatosis, and granulomatous processes such as tuberculosis, and sarcoidosis. Except for papillomatosis, all of the aforementioned conditions may demonstrate hyperattenuation or calcification.

Teaching Points

▶ TPOP is more commonly seen in men, usually over 50 years in age. Most affected patients are asymptomatic.

▶ Higher incidence has been noted in Northern Europe, especially Finland.

▶ TPOP most commonly involves the lower trachea and proximal main bronchi.

▶ On histopathology, multiple, benign submucosal osteocartilaginous nodular growths are seen that maintain a connection with the perichondrium of the cartilaginous rings of the trachea.

▶ CT demonstrates multiple 1- to 5-mm nodular, calcified excrescences, protruding into the airway lumen. The posterior wall of the trachea is spared.

▶ TPOP is not associated with tracheomalacia.

▶ C-ANCA-positive granulomatosis (Wegener) more commonly causes focal nodular wall thickening and luminal narrowing, but rarely can be diffuse.

▶ Coumadin use commonly causes tracheobronchial calcification. The involvement is sometimes patchy, simulating a nodular appearance. However, such calcifications never protrude into the airway lumen and do not cause tracheal wall thickening.

▶ Relapsing polychondritis, similar to TPOP and Coumadin-related airway changes, spares the posterior membrane of the trachea, involves a long segment of the airway, and can calcify. However, relapsing polychondritis causes smooth wall thickening and luminal narrowing and is commonly associated with tracheomalacia.

Management

▶ Treatment is palliative and includes mechanical measures to remove obstructing nodules using cryotherapy, laser excision, external beam irradiation, radiotherapy, stent insertion, or surgical resection therapy.

Further Reading

Javidan-Nejad C. MDCT of trachea and main bronchi. *Radiol Clin North Am*. 2010 Jan;48(1):157-176.

Willms H, Wiechmann V, Sack U, et al. Tracheobronchopathia osteochondroplastica: A rare cause of chronic cough with haemoptysis. *Cough*. 2008 Jun 30;4:4.

History

▶ 27-year-old man presents with shortness of breath.

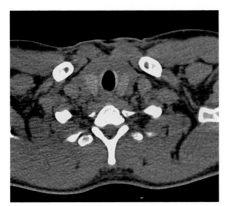
Figure 48.1a

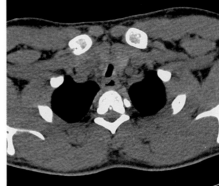
Figure 48.1b

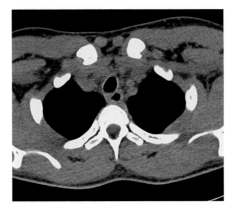
Figure 48.1c

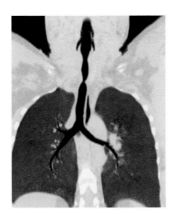
Figure 48.2

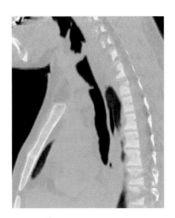
Figure 48.3

Case 48 Short Segment Tracheal Narrowing (from Intubation Injury)

Figure 48.4

Figure 48.5

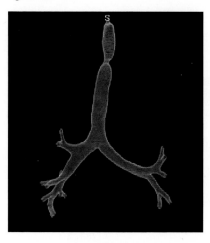

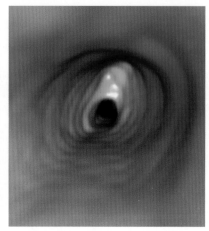

Findings

▶ CT at the level of the thoracic outlet shows a focal stenosis of the trachea and mild asymmetric wall thickening of the right anterolateral wall (Figs. 48.1a–c).

▶ CT reconstruction demonstrates that this wall thickening and luminal narrowing is short and web-like (Fig. 48.2).

▶ Coronal minIP and volume-rendered images confirm the web-like nature of the stenosis (Figs. 48.3–48.5).

Differential Diagnosis

▶ Web-like stenosis at the level of the thoracic outlet is typical of intubation injury. Less likely considerations include granulomatous disease and inhalation injury.

Teaching Points

▶ Post-intubation stenosis remains the most frequent indication for tracheal surgery. It is usually caused by overinflated balloon cuffs or damage from the endotracheal tube tip itself.

▶ The overinflated balloon results in tracheal ischemia and stenosis affecting 360 degrees of the tracheal wall.

▶ Dyspnea on exertion and stridor are the most common presenting symptoms. Patients become symptomatic when the luminal narrowing exceeds 50% of the cross-sectional area.

▶ Focal, concentric or eccentric, web-like wall thickening that protrudes into the lumen can be seen on CT. Findings may be easily overlooked on axial images due to the transverse nature of the web. Coronal and sagittal reconstructions are helpful in detection and characterization.

▶ Tracheostomy injury typically results in collapse of the trachea from left to right as a result of anterior tracheal disruption (akin to removal of a keystone from an arch).

▶ The CT report should include residual luminal diameter, length of the lesion, and the distance of the stenosis from the vocal cords and carina.

Management

▶ Treatment is based on the length and location of the stenosis. It may consist of balloon dilation, laser resection, internal stent, or segmental resection with primary anastomosis.

Further Reading

Grenier PA, Beigelman-Aubry C, Brillet PY. Nonneoplastic tracheal and bronchial stenosis. *Thorac Surg Clin*. 2010 Feb; 20(1):47-64.

Javidan-Nejad C. MDCT of trachea and main bronchi. *Radiol Clin North Am*. 2010 Jan; 48(1):157-176.

History

▶ 57-year-old man with repeated episodes of bronchitis presents for evaluation.

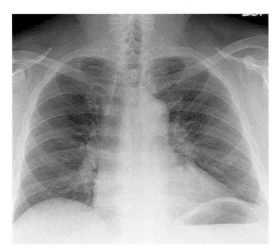

Figure 49.1

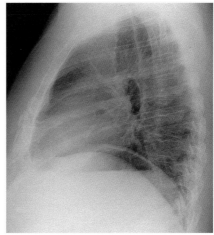

Figure 49.2

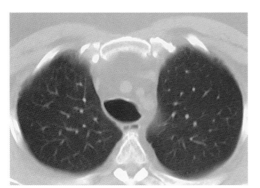

Figure 49.3

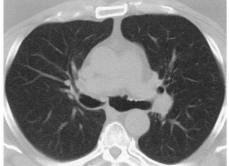

Figure 49.4

Case 49 Tracheobronchomegaly (Mounier-Kuhn)

Figure 49.5

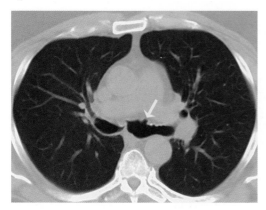

Figure 49.6

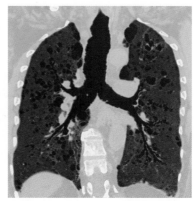

Findings

▶ Chest radiograph (Figs. 49.1 and 49.2) shows enlarged trachea and mainstem bronchi.

▶ CT shows the lemon-shaped trachea (Fig. 49.3). There are focal outpouchings along the bronchial wall (arrow in Fig. 49.5).

▶ Coronal minIP of a different patient with the same disease (Fig. 49.6) shows markedly enlarged trachea and main bronchi, lower lobe and diffuse cystic changes in the lungs. Corrugated contour of the tracheal and bronchial wall is again demonstrated.

Differential Diagnosis

▶ Tracheobronchomegaly can be seen with fibrosis(traction tracheomegaly in severe upper lobe fibrosis) or idiopathic/ congenital tracheobronchomegaly (Mounier-Kuhn [MK]).

Teaching Points

▶ MK is a rare disease affecting the trachea and bronchi.

▶ MK may be associated with generalized elastosis in children, and Ehlers-Danlos and Marfan syndromes in adults.

▶ MK is not associated with smoking.

▶ On pathology, absence or thinning of the muscle, cartilage, and elastic tissue of the airway wall is seen. This leads to uniform dilatation of the trachea and the bronchi of the first to third order.

▶ Conventional radiography demonstrates increased caliber of the trachea, right mainstem bronchi, and left mainstem bronchi exceeding 3 cm, 2.4 cm, and 2.3 cm, respectively.

▶ The inherent structural abnormality of the airway wall causes diverticula to form between the cartilage rings of the trachea and bronchi, creating a corrugated contour of the trachea.

▶ Tracheomalacia is a typical feature of MK seen on both bronchoscopy and CT. On inspiration CT, the trachea can take on a lemon shape. On expiration, collapse of the trachea and bronchi is seen.

▶ Symptoms of MK include chronic cough, increased sputum that clears poorly with coughing, and repeated pneumonias.

▶ The repeated pneumonias lead to bronchiectasis worse in the lower lungs.

▶ Tracheobronchomalacia of various causes can also result in a lemon-shaped trachea. However, unlike MK, there is no increased caliber of the central airways and the diverticulosis of the airway wall is absent.

Management

▶ The central and diffuse nature of this disease precludes surgical management.

▶ Physiotherapy can help clear airway secretions.

Further Reading

Javidan-Nejad C, Bhalla S. Bronchiectasis. *Thorac Clin North Am.* 2010 Feb; 20(1):85-102.

History

▶ 66-year-old woman with new tachycardia and palpitations presents for CT.

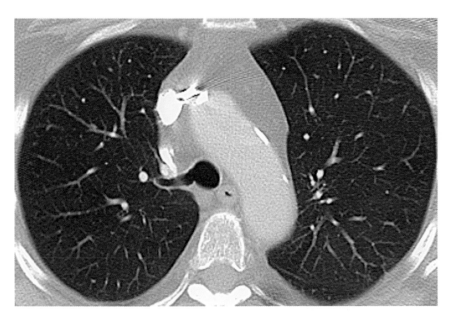

Figure 50.1

Case 50   Tracheal Bronchus

Figure 50.2

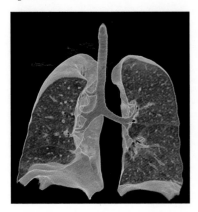

Findings

▸ CT (Fig. 50.1) shows a small bronchus arising from the right lateral wall of the trachea, above the level of the carina.
▸ Volume-rendered image (Fig. 50.2) shows its relationship superior to the right mainstem bronchus.

Differential Diagnosis

▸ Accessory bronchus leads the differential diagnosis. Another, less likely possibility would include a tracheal diverticulum, which does not have a discernible cartilaginous wall and fails to branch in the lung parenchyma.

Teaching Points

▸ A tracheal bronchus is an aberrant bronchus arising from the trachea, anywhere proximal to the origin of the normal upper lobe bronchus. The tracheal bronchus is directed to the upper lobes of either lung and provides airflow to part of the upper lobe or the whole lobe.
▸ In 25% of patients with a tracheal bronchus, the airway is considered a supernumerary bronchus, in which the normal upper lobe bronchus has a typical branching pattern. In the remaining 75% of patients, the tracheal bronchus is considered a displaced bronchus because it is the only air supply to the upper lobe segment.
▸ The overall incidence of right-sided tracheal bronchus is 0.1% to 2% and that of left-sided tracheal bronchus is 0.3% to 1%. In 6% to 9% of cases they are bilateral.
▸ If arising from the trachea, they occur between 2 and 6 cm above the trachea.
▸ A pig bronchus or *bronchus suis* is a subtype of tracheal bronchus in which the entire right upper lobe bronchus is displaced and arises from the trachea.
▸ A tracheal lobe is present when there is an accessory fissure separating the portion of the lung aerated by the tracheal bronchus.
▸ Usually tracheal bronchi are asymptomatic. Symptoms are more common with the left-sided and supernumerary types. Symptoms include recurrent infections, cough, and stridor and occur when there is an abnormal angle or origin of the bronchus, causing poor aeration or drainage.
▸ Obstruction during endotracheal intubation can cause right upper lobe atelectasis.
▸ Diagnosis is made by identifying the abnormal bronchus on various imaging modalities. Coronal reconstruction and volume-rendered reformation of CT data can effectively display the abnormal branching pattern.

Management

▸ No treatment is required. This is a normal variant.

Further Reading

Desir A, Ghaye B. Congenital abnormalities of intrathoracic airways. *Radiol Clin North Am.* 2009 Mar;47(2):203-225.

Part 5   Esophageal Cases

History

► 21-year-old man complains of chest pressure after eating.

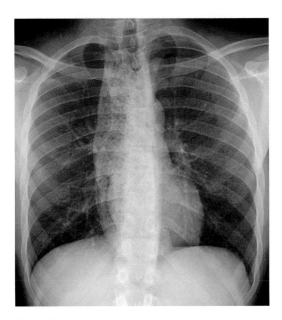

Figure 51.1

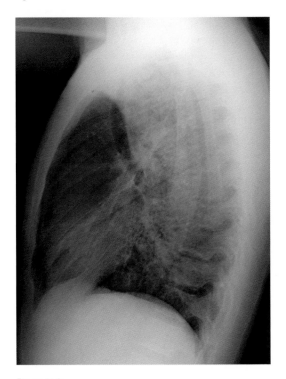

Figure 51.2

Case 51 Achalasia

Figure 51.3

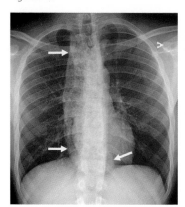

Figure 51.4

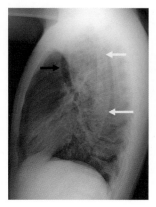

Figure 51.5

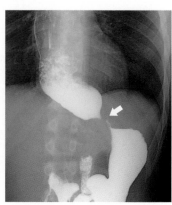

Findings

▶ Chest radiograph shows a tubular soft tissue density mass (white arrows in Figs. 51.3 and 51.4) with mottled air extending through the middle mediastinum from the thoracic inlet to the diaphragm. The trachea is deviated anteriorly (black arrow in Fig. 51.4).

▶ Upper gastrointestinal study confirms the marked dilatation of a debris-filled esophagus with beak-like tapering (thick white arrow in Fig. 51.5) at the gastroesophageal junction. Intermittent emptying of the esophagus into the stomach was noted at the time of the exam, as well as tertiary contractions.

Differential Diagnosis

▶ The chest radiograph finding can only be explained by esophageal dilatation, the differential for which consists of achalasia, a distal esophageal stricture, or an obstructing esophageal or gastric mass. The demonstration of intermittent opening on fluoroscopy and the beak-like tapering would support the diagnosis of achalasia. Occasionally, scleroderma may result in a patulous esophagus, which does not usually reach such a large size.

Teaching Points

▶ A primary esophageal disorder of unclear etiology, achalasia results from destruction of the myenteric plexus, which impairs normal esophageal peristalsis and lower esophageal sphincter function. This results in progressive retention of food products and fluid within the esophagus.

▶ On barium swallow, there is absence of primary and secondary esophageal peristalsis and smooth tapering of the esophagus at the gastroesophageal junction with intermittent relaxation. Esophageal manometry is considered the gold standard for diagnosis.

▶ Rarely, Chagas disease can result in a radiographic appearance similar to achalasia.

▶ Achalasia is associated with a higher rate of nontuberculous mycobacterial infection.

Management

▶ A range of treatment options exist, including balloon dilatation, oral medications, botulinum toxin injection, and surgical myotomy. Referral to a gastroenterologist or surgeon is often indicated.

Further Reading

Franquet T, Erasmus JJ, Gimenez A, Rossi S, Prats R. The retrotracheal space: normal anatomic and pathologic appearances. *Radiographics*. 2002;22:S231-246.

Pohl D, Tutuian R. Achalasia: an overview of diagnosis and treatment. *J Gastrointestin Liver Dis.* 2007 Sep;16(3):297-303.

History

▶ 62-year-old is admitted with acute respiratory failure and sepsis.

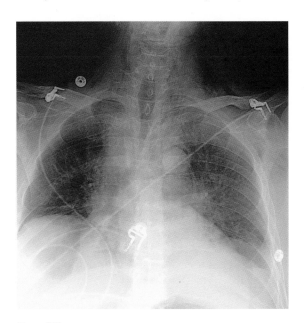

Figure 52.1

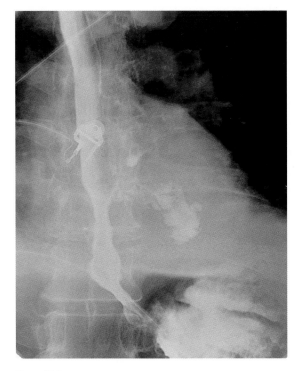

Figure 52.2

Case 52   Esophageal Perforation

Figure 52.3

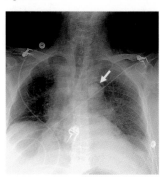

Figure 52.4

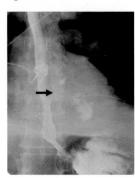

Figure 52.5

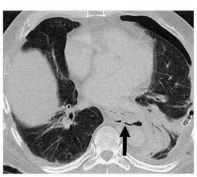

Findings

▶ The chest radiograph demonstrates pneumomediastinum (white arrow in Fig. 52.3) with retrocardiac consolidation and lack of distinction of the descending aorta.

▶ The esophogram demonstrates extravasation of contrast in the lower third of the esophagus, consistent with a leak (black arrow in Fig. 52.4).

▶ Subsequent CT confirms perforation of the esophagus. Discontinuity of the wall of the esophagus with pneumomediastinum and left lower lobe pneumonia are seen. Chest tubes were placed because of suspicion for empyema.

Differential Diagnosis

▶ Based on the differential diagnosis of pneumomediastinum in the absence of trauma, the differential diagnosis would include esophageal perforation, tracheal injury, retroperitoneal gas (from diverticular disease), and spontaneous pneumomediastinum. The left lower lobe pneumonia and small effusion would raise the concern for esophageal perforation, which was confirmed on fluoroscopy.

Teaching Points

▶ Esophageal perforation may occur in a variety of iatrogenic settings: therapeutic endoscopic procedures such as stricture dilation, stent placement, or thermal injury in left atrial radiofrequency ablation.

▶ Esophageal rupture may occur spontaneously, as in Boerhaave syndrome, in which incomplete cricopharyngeal relaxation during vomiting results in abruptly increased intraluminal pressure sufficient to rupture the esophagus.

▶ The distal left posterior wall is the most common site of spontaneous rupture, which classically results in pneumomediastinum and left pleural effusion.

▶ Other possible causes of esophageal perforation include foreign body impaction, caustic and infectious esophagitis, Barrett syndrome, and esophageal cancer.

▶ A dreaded complication of esophageal perforation is the development of mediastinitis, which can be lethal, but can also result in discitis and fistula formation, most notably with the aorta.

▶ Although spontaneous pneumomediastinum may present with chest discomfort, this condition should not present with consolidation or effusions.

Management

▶ The optimal treatment of esophageal perforation depends on a host of considerations. Treatment methods range from nonsurgical management to esophagectomy or surgical exclusion and diversion; however, with an early diagnosis of uncontained perforation, surgery remains the mainstay of therapy.

Further Reading

Fadoo F, Ruiz D, Dawn S, Webb W. Helical CT esophagography for the evaluation of suspected esophageal perforation or rupture. *AJR Am J Roentgenol.* 2004;182:1177-1179.

Young CA, Menias CO, Bhalla S, Prasad SR. CT features of esophageal emergencies. *Radiographics.* 2008 Oct;28(6):1541-1553.

History

▶ 52-year-old woman with chest pain begins her workup with a chest radiograph.

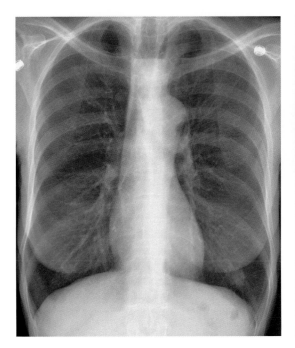

Figure 53.1

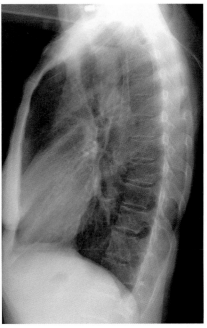

Figure 53.2

Case 53 Esophageal Cancer (with Opacification of the Retrotracheal Triangle)

Figure 53.3

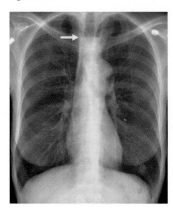

Figure 53.4

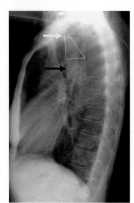

Figure 53.5

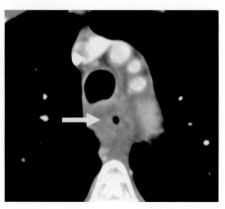

Findings

▶ Air-fluid level (white arrows in Figs. 53.3 and 53.4) is noted in the proximal thoracic esophagus, and mass effect on the posterior wall of the trachea (black arrow in Fig. 53.4) is seen.

▶ CT shows a mid-esophageal circumferential mass (arrow in Fig. 53.5).

Differential Diagnosis

▶ The chest radiograph shows a dilated proximal esophagus, the differential for which includes esophageal neoplasm or middle esophageal stricture. Achalasia could be considered but should not be favored as the distal esophagus is not dilated. The location of the air-fluid level is not typical of an esophageal or Zenker's diverticulum.

Teaching Points

▶ Air-fluid levels encountered in the mediastinum should prompt consideration of esophageal pathology.

▶ Increased opacity in the retrotracheal triangle (triangle in Fig. 53.4) can be seen with esophageal masses, vascular abnormalities such as aberrant subclavian artery, double aortic arch, or aneurysm, and mediastinal extension from a thyroid goiter.

▶ Esophageal cancer has a relatively poor prognosis given its frequent advanced stage at presentation and the lack of a serosal barrier in the esophagus, which allows for mediastinal spread. Loss of the normal fat planes and mass effect on adjacent mediastinal structures is suggestive of direct invasion.

▶ Smoking and alcohol use increase the risk of malignancy, especially squamous cell carcinomas. Adenocarcinomas are usually seen in the setting of gastroesophageal reflux and Barrett's esophagitis.

▶ Esophageal leiomyomas and duplication cysts may mimic malignancies but are smoothly marginated lesions on CT.

Management

▶ The radiographic findings in this case should prompt evaluation of the esophagus by barium swallow or direct endoscopy. If a mass is encountered, CT is used in conjunction with endoscopic ultrasound for staging.

▶ Tumors without mediastinal invasion or distant metastatic disease are surgically resected, usually with gastric pull-through, with or without preoperative chemotherapy.

Further Reading

Franquet T, Erasmus JJ, Gimenez A, et al. The retrotracheal space: normal anatomic and pathologic appearances. *Radiographics*. 2002 Oct;22 Spec No:S231-246.

Noh HM, Fishman EK, Forasteire AA, et al. CT of the esophagus: spectrum of disease with emphasis on esophageal carcinoma. *Radiographics*. 1995 Sep;15(5):1113-1134.

History

▶ 45-year-old woman underwent preoperative chest radiograph prior to hysterectomy.

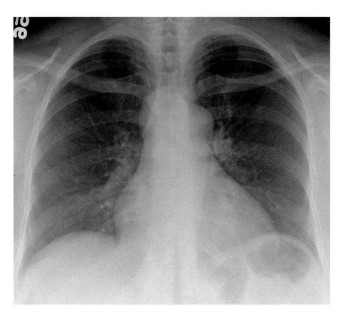

Figure 54.1

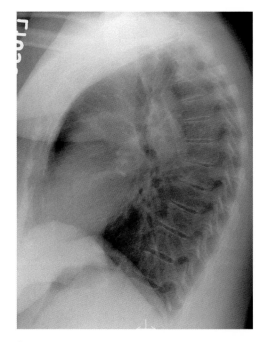

Figure 54.2

Case 54 Esophageal Leiomyoma

Figure 54.3

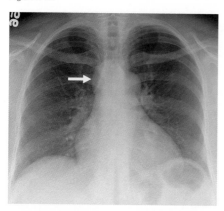

Figure 54.4

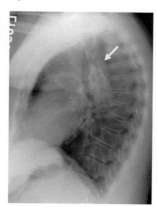

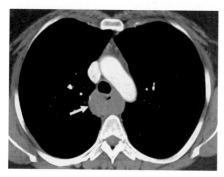

Figure 54.5

Findings

▶ Within the retrotracheal triangle, there is a rounded mass (arrows in Figs. 54.3 and 54.4) that extends above the aortic arch and into the right middle mediastinum.

▶ CT demonstrates a smoothly marginated soft tissue mass (arrow in Fig. 54.5) within the esophageal wall but without evidence of mediastinal fat invasion or tracheal invasion.

Differential Diagnosis

▶ The filling in of the retrotracheal triangle on radiography may be from an esophageal neoplasm, duplication cyst, lymphadenopathy, vascular anomaly, or aneurysm. The CT and endoscopy show a submucosal mass, which would favor a stromal tumor of the esophagus (leiomyoma, leiomyosarcoma, or gastrointestinal stromal tumor [GIST]). Given the esophageal location and lack of aggressive features, leiomyoma would be favored.

Teaching Points

▶ The most common benign esophageal tumors, esophageal leiomyomas, are encapsulated masses of fibrous tissue and smooth muscle fibers that form in the submucosa.

▶ These tumors usually grow slowly and do not tend to cause symptoms until they become large enough to exert mass effect or cause dysphagia. They occur in the middle and distal esophagus but are rare in the upper esophagus, which contains skeletal muscle as opposed to smooth muscle.

▶ As these lesions are submucosal and rarely ulcerate, barium swallows and endoscopy demonstrate normal mucosa overlying the mass.

140

▶ Other submucosal esophageal lesions include GISTs, which arise from the interstitial cells of Cajal, and leiomyosarcomas, which tend to be larger and more aggressive.

Management

▶ As esophageal carcinoma cannot be entirely excluded based on imaging appearance alone, endoscopy with biopsy is required. Surgical resection is performed in all symptomatic patients and is usually performed in asymptomatic patients due to the theoretical risk of symptomatic or malignant transformation.

Further Reading

Jang KM, Lee KS, Lee SJ, et al. The spectrum of benign esophageal lesions: imaging findings. *Korean J Radiol.* 2002 Jul-Sep;3(3): 199-210.

Lee LS, Singhal S, Brinster CJ, et al. Current management of esophageal leiomyoma. *J Am Coll Surg.* 2004 Jan;198(1):136-146.

Part 6   **Pleural Disease**

History

► 73-year-old patient with history of pneumonia presents with persistent fever and elevated white blood cell count.

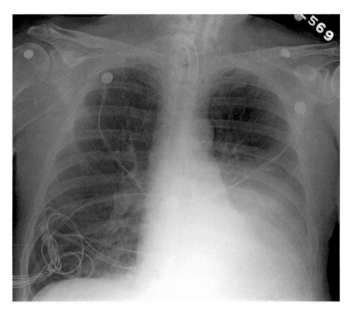

Figure 55.1

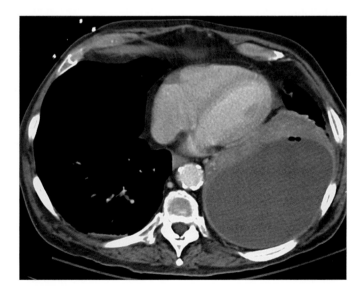

Figure 55.2

Case 55   Empyema

Figure 55.3

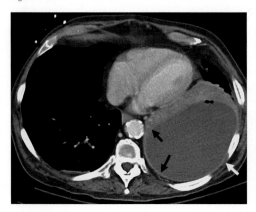

Figure 55.4

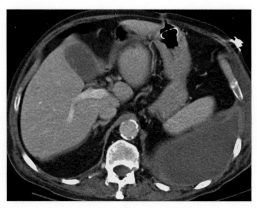

Findings

▶ Chest radiograph (Fig. 55.1) demonstrates a moderate-sized left pleural effusion.

▶ CT demonstrates the effusion with bubbles of gas. Smooth thickening and enhancement of the visceral and parietal pleura consistent with a "split pleura" sign (black arrows in Fig. 55.3) and subpleural edema (white arrow in Fig. 55.3) are seen. The thickening is even easier to see on a more caudal image (Fig. 55.4).

Differential Diagnosis

▶ The differential diagnosis for a unilateral medium pleural effusion is lead by hemothorax, empyema, parapneumonic effusion, and malignancy. When pleural thickening is identified, malignancy and empyema become the major two considerations. The presence of subpleural edema favors empyema.

Teaching Points

▶ Empyema refers to pus in the pleural space. Most often this occurs in the setting of a pneumonia. Empyema connotes a fibropurulent phase, as opposed to a simple exudative parapneumonic effusion.

▶ The split pleura sign is indicative of a complex pleural effusion. In the setting of a smooth pleural surface one would favor an empyema in the differential.

▶ The split pleura sign is seen in about 50% of cases of empyema. Isolated parietal pleura enhancement is also seen in about 50% of cases.

▶ Nodular pleural thickening raises the concern for malignancy, such as mesothelioma or metastatic disease.

▶ An empyema can be distinguished from a lung abscess based on shape, as the empyema tends to be lenticular and assumes different dimensions in different axes. Pulmonary abscesses tend to be spherical, having nearly the same dimension in the sagittal, transverse, and coronal planes.

▶ Gas in the pleural space may be seen in the setting of an empyema, recent intervention, or bronchopleural fistula.

▶ Occasionally, an empyema can break through the chest wall. This is known as an empyema necessitans and can be seen in the setting of tuberculosis, nocardia, and actinomycosis empyema.

Management

▶ Initial management consists of obtaining cultures of the pleural fluid and placing a chest tube for evacuation.

▶ An empyema may become organized and create a rind that restricts lung expansion. This is known as a trapped lung and requires decortication.

Further Reading

Kraus GJ. The split pleura sign. *Radiology*. 2007 Apr;243(1):297-298.

History

▶ 53-year-old man presents with chest pain.

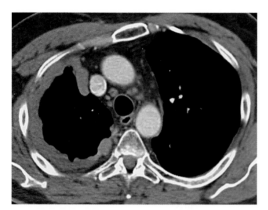

Figure 56.1

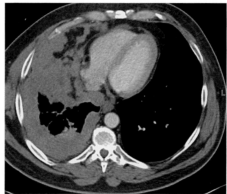

Figure 56.2

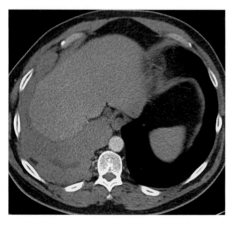

Figure 56.3

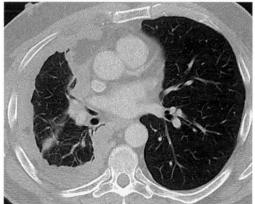

Figure 56.4

Case 56 Malignant Mesothelioma

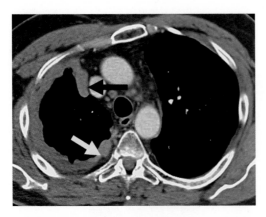

Figure 56.5

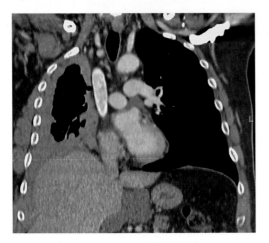

Figure 56.6

Findings

▶ CT with contrast (Figs. 56.1–56.4) shows nodular pleural thickening of the right hemothorax, which is clearly smaller than the left. Note the medial pleural involvement (black arrow in Fig. 56.5) and the nodular extension into the subpleural fat (white arrow in Fig. 56.5). No edema is noted within the subpleural fat.

▶ Coronal reconstruction (Fig. 56.6) shows the extensive pleural involvement and the asymmetry of the lung volumes.

Differential Diagnosis

▶ Pleural thickening can be seen in the setting of infection (empyema), fibrous plaque, or neoplasm. When the thickening is nodular, neoplasm is higher on the differential list and consists of primary tumors (mesothelioma, fibrous tumor of the pleura) or metastatic disease (usually adenocarcinomas). Given the diffuse nodularity and lack of subpleural edema, we would favor mesothelioma or metastases.

Teaching Points

▶ Metastatic disease represents the most common pleural malignancy. Metastases are usually from adenocarcinomas, such as lung, breast, colon, renal, gastric, or colon. Drop metastases to the pleura may be seen in the setting of thymomas and lymphomas.

- Mesothelioma is the most common primary pleural malignancy.
- Signs that are relatively specific for a diagnosis of malignancy include circumferential pleural thickening, nodular pleural thickening, pleural thickening greater than 1 cm, and involvement of the mediastinal pleural surface.
- Absence of pleural nodules does not exclude malignancy in the setting of an exudative effusion.
- Unlike empyema, malignancy rarely results in subpleural edema. Instead, nodular extension into the subpleural fat may be seen, resembling a stalactite.
- Greater than 80% of patients with mesothelioma have had exposure to asbestos. Amphibole fibers (crocidolite and amosite) carry a stronger association with mesothelioma induction, which is postulated to be due to their long, thin shape and greater irritant effect.
- Asbestos exposure is associated with a number of occupations, including insulation manufacturing, mining, sheet metal work, ship fitting, plumbing, and construction.
- Pleural plaques and other findings of asbestos exposure, which were absent in this case, can be used to suggest mesothelioma over metastatic disease.

Management

- Mesothelioma has a very poor prognosis, with a mean survival of <1 year. Chemotherapy alone has not proven to be a successful treatment strategy. Surgery provides the only potential for cure and consists of an extrapleural pneumonectomy (consisting of visceral and parietal pleura, portions of pericardium, and diaphragm). Surgery is reserved for those few patients without metastases or extension to the chest wall or mediastinum.

Further Reading

Dynes MC, White EM, Fry WA, Ghahremani GG. Imaging manifestations of pleural tumors. *Radiographics*. 1992 Nov;12(6):1191-1201.
Salahudeen HM, Hoey ET, Robertson RJ, Darby MJ. CT appearances of pleural tumours. *Clin Radiol*. 2009 Sep;64(9):918-930.

History

▶ 64-year-old man presents with cough and ankle pain.

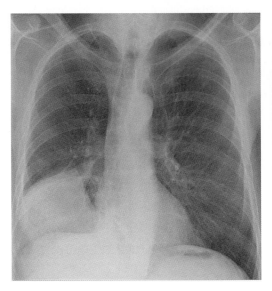

Figure 57.1

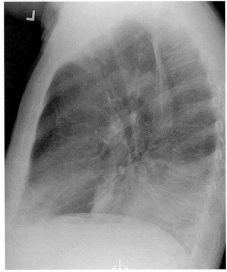

Figure 57.2

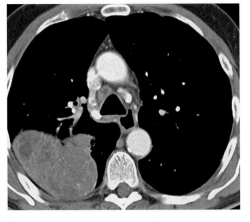

Figure 57.3

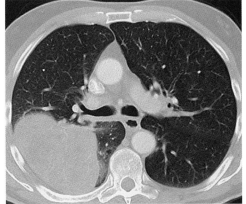

Figure 57.4

Case 57   Fibrous Tumor of the Pleura

Figure 57.5

Figure 57.6

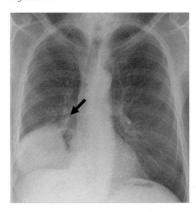
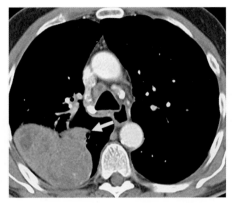

Findings

▶ Initial radiograph shows a right lower opacity with a tail that suggests an intrapleural or fissural location (arrow in Fig. 57.5).
▶ CT confirms the fissural location (arrow in Fig. 57.6). The mass is heterogeneously enhancing, but does not invade any adjacent structures.

Differential Diagnosis

▶ The differential diagnosis is based on the suspicion of a pleural soft tissue mass and includes mesothelioma, metastasis (usually from adenocarcinomas, including lung, breast, renal, and gastrointestinal tract), and fibrous tumor of the pleura (FTP). Other pleural-based masses, such as lipoma and plaque, would not be so heterogeneous and large. The large size, heterogeneity, and lack of primary tumor would favor FTP.

Teaching Points

▶ FTPs are unusual pleural tumors that are not associated with asbestos exposure.
▶ They are believed to arise from submesothelial connective tissue. Because the cell of origin is not mesothelial, the term *benign mesothelioma* is not accurate.
▶ FTPs are distinguished from malignant mesothelioma by their morphology (often pedunculated), histology, immunohistochemistry, and radiologic appearance.
▶ Because up to 20% of FTPs may be aggressive with more malignant features, the term *benign* fibrous tumor is usually avoided.
▶ Usually, FTPs are asymptomatic and discovered incidentally on chest radiography.
▶ Extrathoracic manifestations reported in the literature include hypertrophic osteoarthropathy, clubbing, hypoglycemia (from an insulin-like hormone), and galactorrhea (from a prolactin-like hormone).
▶ The role of FDG-PET in these lesions has yet to be determined. Early work suggests these tumors show some uptake but are not as FDG-avid as malignant mesothelioma.

Management

▶ All FTPs are completely resected. Percutaneous biopsy cannot reliably exclude malignancy because of frequent intratumoral hypocellular areas, which may lead to sampling error.
▶ Should they recur, repeat excision or radiofrequency ablation is recommended.

Further Reading

Rosado-de-Christenson ML, Abbott GF, McAdams HP, et al. From the archives of the AFIP: Localized fibrous tumors of the pleura. *Radiographics*. 2003;23:759-783.

History

▶ 83-year-old man presents with cough.

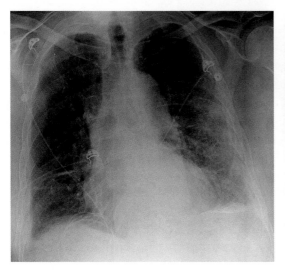

Figure 58.1

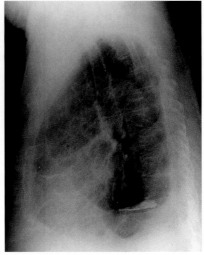

Figure 58.2

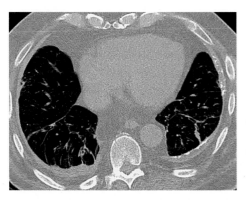

Figure 58.3

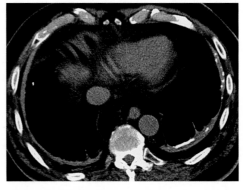

Figure 58.4

Case 58   Pleural Plaques (from Asbestos Exposure)

Figure 58.5

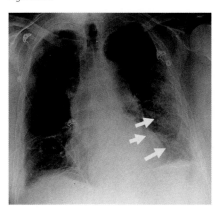

Figure 58.6

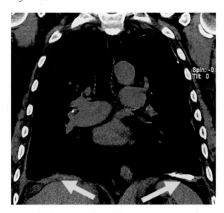

Findings

▸ Chest radiograph (Figs. 58.1 and 58.2) demonstrates lower-lobe-predominant pleural thickening over the diaphragm.

▸ On the frontal radiograph, a vague opacity is seen overlying the left lower lobe. The right margin is scalloped (arrows in Fig. 58.5). This appearance has been referred to as the holly-leaf sign and is characteristic of pleural plaquing, as is absence of visualization of the opacity on the lateral.

▸ CT (Figs. 58.3 and 58.4) shows uniform pleural thickening with calcification. No parenchymal abnormalities are seen.

▸ Coronal reconstruction (Fig. 58.6) better demonstrates the pleural plaques on the diaphragm (white arrows). There is relative sparing of the costophrenic angle and no involvement of the apices.

Differential Diagnosis

▸ Based on the chest radiograph, calcified plaque is seen on the left. The differential diagnosis includes plaquing from asbestos exposure, prior empyema, or trauma (hemothorax). Once noncalcified plaque is seen on the right, asbestos exposure must head the list.

Teaching Points

▸ When unilateral pleural plaques (thickening) are seen, one should consider etiologies other than asbestos exposure, such as prior infection or trauma.

▸ The majority of pleural plaques (90%) are not calcified.

▸ The presence of pleural plaques in the setting of asbestos exposure is not necessarily asbestosis. *Asbestosis* is pulmonary fibrosis in the setting of asbestos exposure.

▸ Pleural plaques that involve the posterior lateral wall, the sixth to ninth ribs laterally, the dome of the diaphragm, and the mediastinal surface are almost diagnostic of pleural plaques from asbestos exposure.

▸ Pleural plaques should be uniform in their thickness. More mass-like areas should be approached with caution, as patients with asbestos exposure have a higher incidence of lung cancer and mesothelioma.

Management

▸ CT is the most sensitive modality for the diagnosis of pleural plaques.

▸ Pleural plaques are benign and do not require treatment or follow-up.

Further Reading

Kim KI, Kim CW, Lee MK, et al. Imaging of occupational lung disease. *Radiographics*. 2001;21(6);1371-1391.

Roach HD, Davies GJ, Attanoos R, et al. Asbestos: when the dust settles: an imaging review of asbestos-related disease. *Radiographics*. 2002;22 Spec No:S167-184.

History

▶ 54-year-old man with a history of lung cancer presents with a persistent pneumothorax after thoracentesis.

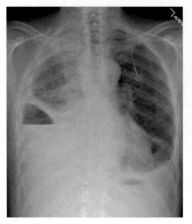

Figure 59.1

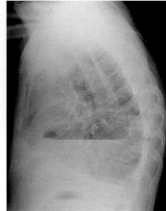

Figure 59.2

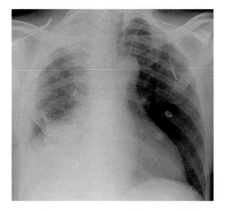

Figure 59.3

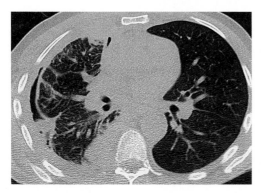

Figure 59.4

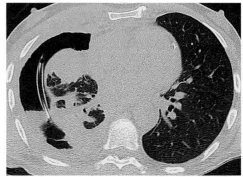

Figure 59.5

Case 59 Trapped Lung (from Pleural Metastases)

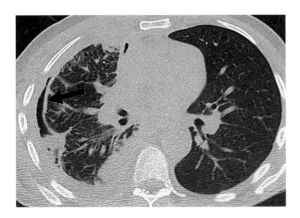

Figure 59.6

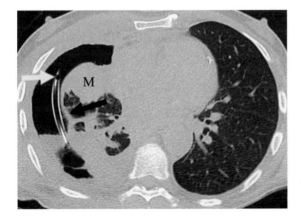

Figure 59.7

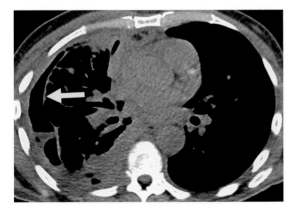

Figure 59.8

Findings

▶ Chest radiograph (Figs. 59.1–59.3) shows a moderate-sized hydropneumothorax that does not change after chest tube placement (Fig. 59.3). Mediastinal lymphadenopathy and interstitial opacities were known to represent metastases.

▶ CT shows pleural thickening (black arrows in Figs. 59.6 and 59.7) that is so pronounced that the pleura can be seen on soft tissue windows (white arrow in Fig. 59.8).

▶ Despite adequate placement of the chest tube (white arrow in Fig. 59.7 represents the side hole of the thoracostomy tube), the hydropneumothorax persists. (M in Fig. 59.7 = the primary cancer.)

Differential Diagnosis

▶ If a pneumothorax persists after chest tube placement, one must consider chest tube malfunction, air leak (bronchopleural fistula or bronchial fracture), or inability for the lung to expand (trapped or drowned lung). The visualization of the thickened pleura allows for the diagnosis of trapped lung.

Teaching Points

▶ Post-thoracentesis pneumothorax is a well-known complication that usually arises from a pleural tear.

▶ Occasionally, hydropneumothorax after thoracentesis will be a manifestation of the inability of the lung to expand. When the lung fails to expand as a result of mucus plug or central mass, the term *drowned lung* is used. If the lung fails to expand because of a constrictive pleural peel, it is known as a *trapped lung*.

▶ Treatment consists of relieving the obstruction (removing the central plug or mass in a drowned lung or decortication for a trapped lung). Placement of a chest tube does not treat the hydropneumothorax.

▶ Trapped lung may be from empyema, chronic inflammation, hemothorax, or malignancy.

▶ The term *pneumothorax ex vacuo* was originally used to describe a spontaneous pneumothorax in the setting of lobar collapse (usually right upper lobe). Increasingly, this term is used to describe a pneumothorax from a drowned or trapped lung.

Management

▶ If a trapped lung is from a benign condition, decortication is considered, but if it is from malignancy, treatment is mainly palliative as the prognosis is very poor (6-month mean survival).

Further Reading

Huggins JT, Doelken P, Sahn SA. The unexpandable lung. *F1000 Med Rep.* 2010;2:77.

Part 7 Chest Wall Cases

History

▶ 32-year-old man with a palpable axillary mass presents for preoperative imaging.

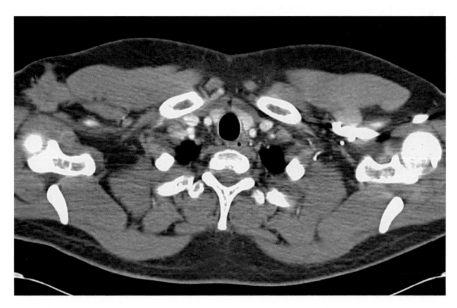

Figure 60.1

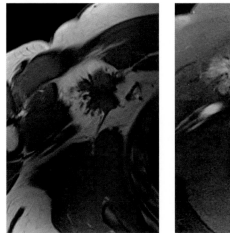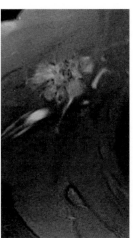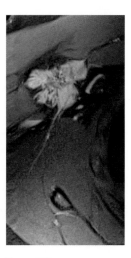

Figure 60.2a   Figure 60.2b   Figure 60.2c

Case 60   Desmoid Tumor

Figure 60.3

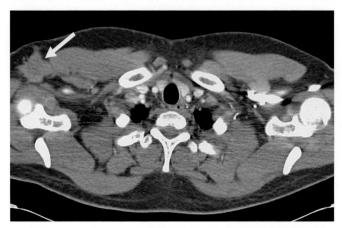

Findings

▶ Spiculated mass in the right axilla which is iso-attenuating with adjacent musculature on CT (arrow in Fig. 60.3)
▶ On MR, the lesion has signal intensity equal to muscle on T1-weighted image (Fig. 60.2a), is higher in signal intensity than muscle on T2-weighted image (Fig. 60.2b), and enhances with gadolinium (Fig. 60.2c).

Differential Diagnosis

▶ The differential comprises desmoid tumor (fibromatosis), lymphoma, matted lymphadenopathy, sarcoma, or metastases. Given the lack of a primary tumor and the patient's young age, desmoid tumor would be favored.

Teaching Points

▶ Desmoid tumors are fibroblastic/myofibroblastic neoplasms that originate from musculo-aponeurotic structures and are part of the group of conditions known as deep fibromatoses.
▶ Desmoid tumors are often seen in the chest wall, most frequently in the soft tissues surrounding the shoulder and axilla.
▶ Desmoid tumors are considered benign by histology but can be locally aggressive. They rarely metastasize.
▶ Desmoid tumors are often associated with young age (<30), female gender, and familial adenomatous polyposis (FAP) and sporadically may occur at sites of previous trauma, scars, or irradiation.
▶ On cross-sectional imaging, desmoid tumors tend to follow the attenuation of adjacent musculature on CT and on T1-weighted MR. In fact, at first glance, the mass can be confused for muscle. Their borders tend to be spiculated. Desmoid tumors tend to be brighter than muscle on T2-weighted imaging and enhance with gadolinium.

Management

▶ Because of its potential to grow and locally infiltrate, radical tumor resection with free margins remains the first therapy of choice. In cases with anatomical or technical limitations for a wide excision, radiation therapy represents a proven and effective alternative or supplementary treatment.
▶ Owing to their infiltrative nature, complete resection with clean margins can prove to be challenging. For larger lesions, a multidisciplinary approach is taken to ensure that the treatment is not worse than the desmoid tumor itself.

Further Reading

Bölke E, Krasniqi H, Lammering G, et al. Chest wall and intrathoracic desmoid tumors: surgical experience and review of the literature. *Eur J Med Res.* 2009 Jun 18;14(6):240-243.
O'Sullivan P, O'Dwyer H, Flint J, et al. Soft tissue tumours and mass-like lesions of the chest wall: a pictorial review of CT and MR findings. *Br J Radiol.* 2007 Jul;80(955):574-580.

History

▶ 66-year-old woman with a history of endometrial and renal carcinoma now presents with elevated tumor markers and a palpable mass inferior to her left scapula.

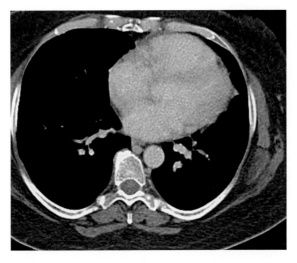

Figure 61.1

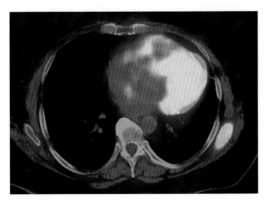

Figure 61.2

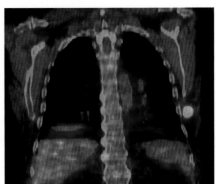

Figure 61.3

Case 61 Elastofibroma Dorsi

Figure 61.4

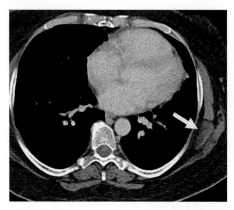

Findings

▶ A low-attenuation mass (arrow in Fig. 61.4) is seen in the soft tissues just medial to the left latissimus dorsi and posterior to the serratus anterior muscle.

▶ On the fused FDG-PET images (Figs. 61.2 and 61.3) the mass shows increased uptake.

Differential Diagnosis

▶ Though metastasis may be considered, the patient's age, the location of the lesion, and the CT attenuation of the lesion are characteristic of elastofibroma dorsi.

Teaching Points

▶ Elastofibroma dorsi is a mass-like condition that represents a proliferation of hyalinized collagen, fibroblasts, and mature adipose tissue. It is not a neoplasm, and unlike desmoid tumor, it does not locally invade or metastasize.

▶ The pathogenesis has been related to a repeated mechanical friction between the chest wall and the scapula.

▶ On CT, elastofibroma dorsi will usually appear as a well-circumscribed mass with lower attenuation than the surrounding muscles. Thin-section CT and MR will show a layering of soft tissue attenuation/intensity with fat, giving the mass a characteristic striated appearance.

▶ Elastofibroma dorsi may be slightly higher than the adjacent muscle on
T2-weighted MR image and usually has minimal enhancement after gadolinium.

▶ As the pathogenesis is believed to be from mechanical stress, elastofibroma dorsi can have increased uptake of FDG on PET.

▶ Elastofibroma dorsi is usually asymptomatic and discovered incidentally by the patient, who notes the mass protruding in the scapular region.

▶ Elastofibroma dorsi is typically found in elderly women (females/males: 13/1).

Management

▶ Imaging studies should provide the definite diagnosis. Rarely, biopsy is performed.

▶ Once the diagnosis is made, no treatment is needed.

Further Reading

Malghem J, Baudrez V, Lecouvet F, et al. Imaging study findings in elastofibroma dorsi. *Joint Bone Spine*. 2004 Nov;71(6):536-541.

O'Sullivan P, O'Dwyer H, Flint J, et al. Soft tissue tumours and mass-like lesions of the chest wall: a pictorial review of CT and MR findings. *Br J Radiol*. 2007 Jul;80(955):574-580.

History

▶ 57-year-old man with history of lymphoma of the parotid gland is worked up for an abnormal admitting chest radiograph.

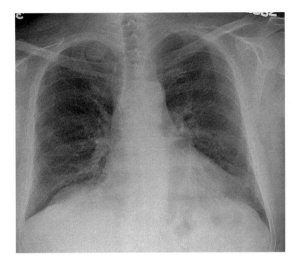

Figure 62.1

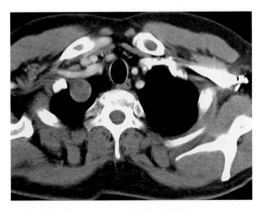

Figure 62.2

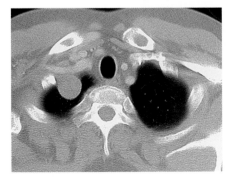

Figure 62.3

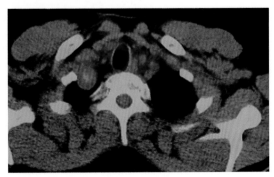

Figure 62.4

Case 62   Extrapulmonary Mass (Schwannoma of the Brachial Plexus)

Figure 62.5

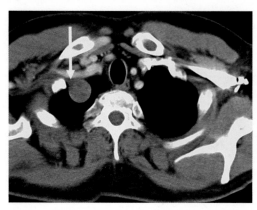

Findings

► Chest radiograph at the time of initial staging shows a well-circumscribed mass in the right upper thorax (Fig. 62.1). There is no correlate on the lateral examination (not shown).

► Subsequent CT (Figs. 62.2 and 62.3) shows a well-defined, rounded mass in the apex. The mass is extrapulmonary and has some low-attenuation regions. It also has some higher-attenuation regions, representing enhancing elements. The mass is contiguous with the brachial plexus (arrow in Fig. 62.5)

► FDG PET-CT, performed for lymphoma staging, shows only mild uptake in the lesion (Fig. 62.4).

Differential Diagnosis

► Although metastases are a concern in a patient with lymphoma, the mass is well rounded and extrapulmonary. This appearance is characteristic of a peripheral nerve sheath tumor. In a patient without neurofibromatosis, the lesion is typical for a schwannoma.

Teaching Points

► Schwannomas and neurofibromas represent nerve sheath tumors that may arise in the intercostal nerves and the brachial plexus.

► Neurofibromas are more commonly seen with neurofibromatosis and have a higher rate of malignant transformation than schwannomas.

► Schwannomas tend to have low-attenuating regions, reflecting the high myelin content.

► Schwannomas may enhance after intravenous contrast on CT. On MR, contrast enhancement is easily seen after gadolinium. The MR appearance has been classically described as a target on T2-weighted imaging with a bright lesion and central low-intensity region (see Case 74).

► Schwannomas may cause adjacent rib erosion, which should not be mistaken for invasion.

► FDG-PET can be useful for staging when the patient is known to have a malignant nerve sheath tumor, but care must be taken in using FDG-PET to evaluate an isolated lesion, as benign nerve sheath tumors may have uptake.

Management

► Imaging allows for a confident diagnosis of schwannoma.

► On occasion, patients may present with chest pain. In these situations, the lesions may be resected to potentially help symptoms and to exclude the remote possibility of a malignant nerve sheath tumor.

Further Reading

Kuhlman JE, Bouchardy L, Fishman EK, Zerhouni EA. CT and MR imaging evaluation of chest wall disorders. *Radiographics*. 1994 May;14(3):571-595.

History

▶ 45-year-old man with shortness of breath undergoes chest radiography.

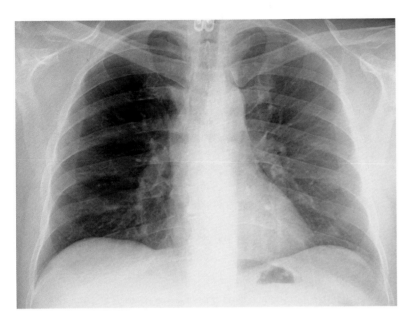

Figure 63.1

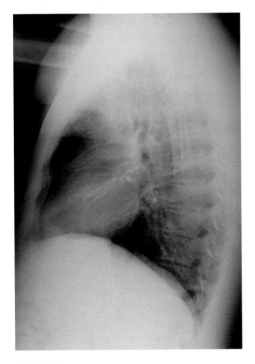

Figure 63.2

Case 63   Poland Syndrome

Figure 63.3

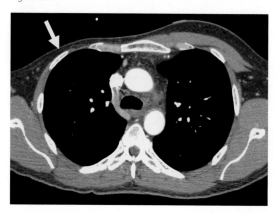

Findings

▶ Hyperlucent right hemithorax is noted on the frontal radiograph (Fig. 63.1) with preserved lung volume and normal vascularity.

▶ Subsequent CT (Fig. 63.3) demonstrates absence of the right pectoralis muscles (arrow) and provides the diagnosis.

Differential Diagnosis

▶ A unilateral hyperlucent lung should prompt one to consider (from outside in) Poland syndrome, mastectomy (in women), anterior pneumothorax (in supine patient), contralateral pleural effusion (supine patient), Swyer-James syndrome, and in children, a radiolucent endobronchial foreign body. Rarely, a large central pulmonary embolism can result in a unilateral hyperlucent lung (Westermark sign). Given that the radiograph is upright, the patient is a man, and pulmonary vascularity and volume are preserved, Poland syndrome should be favored by the radiograph.

Teaching Points

▶ When a hyperlucent hemithorax is encountered, assessment of the volume and vascularity of the lung is necessary in ordering a differential diagnosis. Decreased volume can also be seen in scimitar (congenital hypovenolobar) syndrome and Swyer-James syndrome (obliterative bronchiolitis).

▶ Expiration imaging may show air-trapping of the lucent lung which is typical for Swyer-James syndrome and an endobronchial foreign body.

▶ Chest wall abnormalities can also make the lung appear hyperlucent due to absence of soft tissue structures lessening the density of the affected side. In women, mastectomy changes often produce this appearance.

▶ Poland syndrome is a rare congenital disorder characterized by varying degrees of chest wall hypoplasia and ipsilateral hand abnormalities. The sternal portions of the pectoralis major muscle are absent and varying degrees of rib and costal cartilage hypoplasia are seen. One theory suggests that subclavian artery hypoplasia (or branch vessel hypoplasia) leads to the abnormality. Hand anomalies can occur, most commonly shortness of the middle phalanges and cutaneous webbing.

Management

▶ Depending of the severity of the chest wall deformity, surgical correction may be undertaken with muscle flap transposition and/or bone grafting for chest wall support. In children, this is generally a staged procedure due to ongoing growth and maturation. Surgical intervention may also be undertaken for cosmesis.

Further Reading

Fokin AA, Robicsek F. Poland's syndrome revisited. *Ann Thorac Surg.* 2002 Dec;74(6):2218-2225.
Jeung MY, Gangi A, Gasser B, et al. Imaging of chest wall disorders. *Radiographics.* 1999 May-Jun;19(3):617-637.

History

▶ 72-year-old man is admitted for severe chest pain.

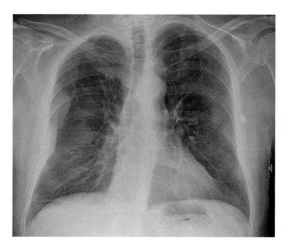

Figure 64.1

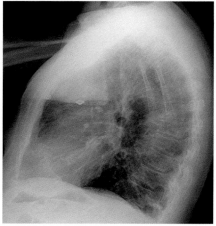

Figure 64.2

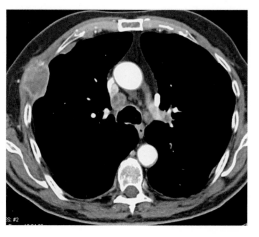

Figure 64.3

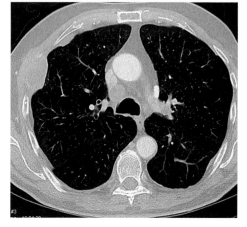

Figure 64.4

Case 64   Chest Wall Metastases (from Lung Cancer)

Figure 64.5

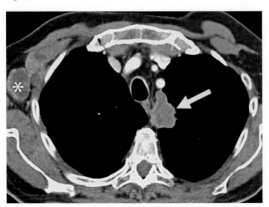

Figure 64.6

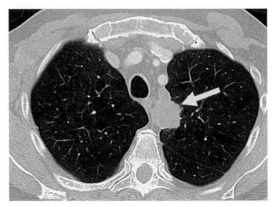

Findings

► Chest radiograph (Figs. 64.1 and 64.2) shows a bilobed pleural/subpleural mass in the right mid-thorax. Another ill-defined opacity is seen slightly more medially. These opacities are hard to see on the lateral, suggesting that they are extrapulmonary. The presence of the incomplete border sign on the frontal radiograph also suggests that the mass is extrapulmonary. The incomplete border sign refers to the clear border with the lung that is seen along the left border but the lack of clear demarcation with the chest wall along the right border.

► CT with contrast (Figs. 64.3 and 64.4) confirms the extrapulmonary nature of the mass. Images at a slightly higher level better show a mass above the aortic arch (arrows in Figs. 64.5 and 64.6) and right axillary lymphadenopathy (asterisk in Fig. 64.5).

Differential Diagnosis

► Chest wall masses may be from metastatic disease, infection, or primary tumors of the chest wall. Given the lung mass and lymphadenopathy, metastatic lung cancer should be favored.

Teaching Points

► Most masses in the chest wall represent metastatic cancer, usually from lung cancer, breast cancer, melanoma, lymphoma, or renal cell cancer.

► Other adenocarcinomas, including colon, prostate, and pancreatic cancers, are well known to metastasize to the ribs and chest wall.

► In an older patient, multiple myeloma may initially present with multiple chest wall masses.

► Primary tumors of the chest wall are not as common as metastases. They include benign entities, such as nerve sheath tumors, desmoid tumors, and lipomas.

► Malignant primary lesions of the chest wall are usually sarcomas, most commonly fibrosarcomas and malignant fibrous histiocytomas (also known as undifferentiated pleomorphic sarcomas).

► Lung infections may break out of the pleura to involve the chest wall as well. Organisms that are well known to present with chest wall involvement include nocardia, actinomycosis, aspergillus, and tuberculosis.

Management

► Chest wall lesions are important to note in the report because they are easily biopsied by ultrasound or CT and are often readily amenable to core biopsy. With one biopsy, a patient can be staged and diagnosed.

Further Reading

Jeung MY, Gangi A, Gasser B, et al. Imaging of chest wall disorders. *Radiographics*. 1999 May-Jun;19(3):617-637.

History

▶ 71-year-old woman with fever receives this radiograph.

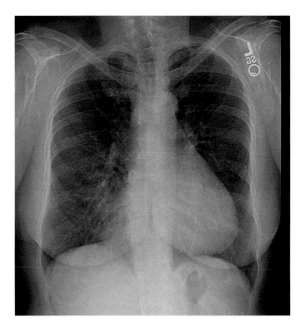

Figure 65.1

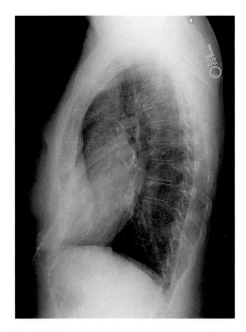

Figure 65.2

Case 65 Pectus Excavatum (Pseudo Right Middle Lobe Pneumonia)

Figure 65.3

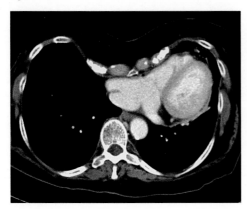

Figure 65.4

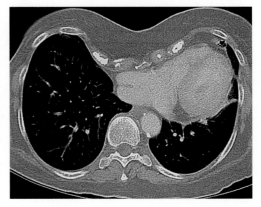

Findings

▶ The right heart border is not well seen on the frontal radiograph (Fig. 65.1), yet no consolidation or collapse is seen in the region of the middle lobe on the lateral projection (Fig. 65.2). Instead, a sternal deformity is seen on the lateral projection.

▶ CT performed in search of an abdominal source of fever (Figs. 65.3 and 65.4) shows the pectus configuration and the adjacent clear right lung.

Differential Diagnosis

▶ Right middle lobe pneumonia without pectus excavatum and clear lungs in the setting of a pectus excavatum are the only two reasonable options. Once the lateral radiograph is seen, only the latter should be offered.

Teaching Points

▶ Pectus excavatum (sometimes referred to as funnel chest) is one of the most common congenital deformities of the sternum.

▶ In this condition, sternal and costochondral depression reduce the anteroposterior dimension of the thorax in the midline, resulting in leftward displacement and rotation of the heart. The normal cardiac borders, then, are not seen on the chest radiograph.

▶ The altered appearance of the right heart border can be confused with the silhouette sign of right middle lobe collapse or pneumonia if the frontal radiograph is viewed alone. The lateral will allow for a confident diagnosis of pectus excavatum.

▶ Frequently, pectus excavatum is associated with thoracic scoliosis.

▶ The severity of the pectus excavatum is best quantified with CT. The pectus index or Haller index can be derived by dividing the transverse diameter of the chest by the anteroposterior diameter.

▶ Haller et al. found the normal value of this index to be 2.56 (±0.35 SD) and suggested that a pectus index >3.25 necessitates surgical correction.

Management

▶ Identification of the pectus excavatum on the lateral should suffice unless the pectus is severe enough to contemplate surgery.

Further Reading

Haller JA, Kramer SS, Lietman SA. Use of CT scans in selection of patients for pectus excavatum surgery: a preliminary report. *J Pediatr Surg.* 1987;10:904-906.
Jeung MY, Gangi A, Gasser B, et al. Imaging of chest wall disorders. *Radiographics.* 1999 May-Jun;19(3):617-637.

Part 8

Mediastinal Vascular Cases

Mediastinal vascular case

History

▶ 62-year-old woman with history of repaired coarctation of aorta receives an infusion catheter placed for treatment of breast cancer.

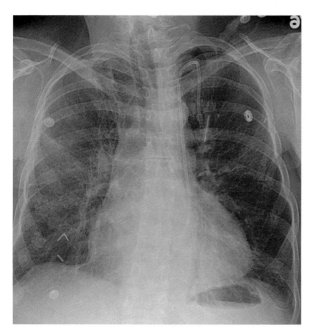

Figure 66.1

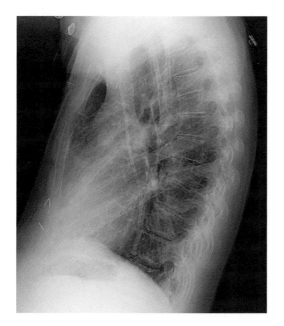

Figure 66.2

Case 66   Catheter in Persistent Left Superior Vena Cava

Figure 66.3a

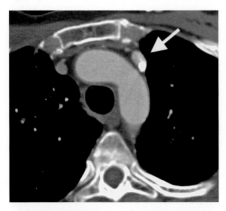

Figure 66.3b

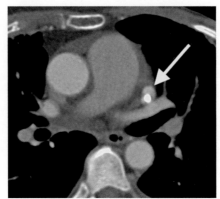

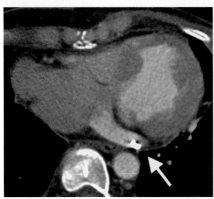

Figure 66.3c

Findings

▶ Radiograph (Figs. 66.1 and 66.2) shows an infusion catheter placed through the left subclavian vein coursing along the left lateral mediastinum, curving toward the midline on the frontal radiograph (Fig. 66.1) and superimposed on the middle mediastinum on the lateral radiograph (Fig. 66.2).

▶ CT confirms the course of the catheter in the left-sided superior vena cava (arrows in Fig. 66.3a–c).

Differential Diagnosis

▶ The differential diagnosis for a catheter traveling along the left mediastinal border includes a catheter in a left-sided superior vena cava (LSVC), left upper lobe partial anomalous pulmonary venous return, left superior intercostal vein, left internal mammary vein, and left pericardiophrenic vein. Given the vertical course on the frontal and the middle mediastinal course on the lateral, LSVC would be favored.

Teaching Points

▶ Persistent LSVC is the most common venous anomaly of the main thoracic veins. It occurs in 0.3% to 0.5% of the general population.

▶ Usually asymptomatic, it is discovered when an attempt is made to access the right heart by placing a central line or pacemaker leads through a left internal jugular or left subclavian venous approach.

- A right-sided SVC is also present in 85% of cases of LSVC. If there is a duplicated SVC, the left brachiocephalic vein may never connect to the right.
- LSVC drains into the coronary sinus and should be suspected when a dilated coronary sinus is found in the absence of right atrial or right ventricular enlargement.

Management

- LSVC draining into an intact coronary sinus does not require treatment.
- LSVC may have implications when percutaneous ablation of atrial arrhythmias is being considered and should be noted in the Radiology report.

Further Reading

Goyal SK, Punnam SR, Verma G, et al. Persistent left superior vena cava: a case report and review of literature. *Cardiovasc Ultrasound.* 2008 Oct 10;6:50.

Webb W, Gamsu G, Speckman J, et al. Computed tomographic demonstration of mediastinal venous anomalies. *AJR Am J Roentgenol.* 1982;139(1):157-161.

History

▶ 57-year-old woman complains of mild dysphagia.

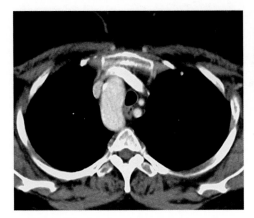

Figure 67.1a

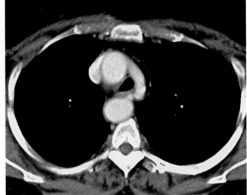

Figure 67.1b

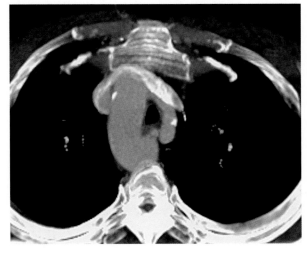

Figure 67.2

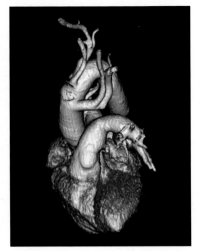

Figure 67.3

Case 67   Double Aortic Arch

Figure 67.4a

Figure 67.4b

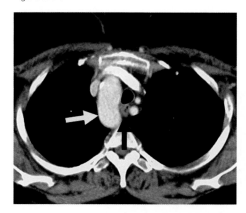
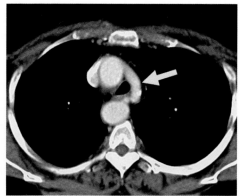

Findings

▶ CT angiography demonstrates two aortic arches: one arch (white arrow in Fig. 67.4a) is right of the trachea at the level of the manubrium and a second one is left of the trachea. Note the esophageal thickening at the same level (black arrow in Fig. 67.4a). The left arch is smaller and more inferior (Fig. 67.4b).

▶ Thick maximum-intensity projection shows the ring created by the two arches on one image (Fig. 67.2). Volume-rendered CT nicely illustrates each arch giving rise to ipsilateral common carotid and subclavian arteries (Fig. 67.3).

Differential Diagnosis

▶ Differential diagnosis consists of aortic arch anomalies and mainly includes double aortic arch, left aortic arch with aberrant right subclavian artery, and right aortic arch with aberrant left subclavian artery.

Teaching Points

▶ Aortic arch anomalies can form vascular rings that cause tracheoesophageal compression. Double aortic arch is the most common vascular ring to cause symptoms. Most patients are asymptomatic, but if symptomatic, they present with dysphagia, stridor, and recurrent infections.

▶ In double aortic arch two arches are present; with the right-sided arch usually larger and more superior than the left-sided arch. Each arch gives rise to its ipsilateral subclavian and carotid arteries.

▶ The descending aorta is usually left-sided.

▶ The distal left-sided arch is occasionally atretic, resulting in a fibrous cord. This cord is usually not directly seen on CT or MR. Because it creates a tight ring, secondary signs, especially tracheal compression, clue the reader to its presence.

▶ The longstanding extrinsic compression of the central airways by the vascular ring can cause tracheobronchomalacia that may persist after surgical repair.

▶ Double aortic arch is not associated with an increased incidence of congenital heart disease.

Management

▶ Symptomatic relief may be achieved with surgical ligation of the nondominant arch.

Further Reading

Chan MS, Chu WC, Cheung KL, et al. Angiography and dynamic airway evaluation with MDCT in the diagnosis of double aortic arch associated with tracheomalacia. *AJR Am J Roentgenol.* 2005 Nov; 185(5):1248-1251.

Türkvatan A, Büyükbayraktar FG, Olçer T, et al. Congenital anomalies of the aortic arch: evaluation with the use of multidetector computed tomography. *Korean J Radiol.* 2009 Mar-Apr;10(2):176-184.

History

▶ 49-year-old man with new left internal jugular catheter presents for a chest radiograph to confirm placement (Fig. 68.1). Incidentally, he has a prior CT of the chest (Figs. 68.2–68.4).

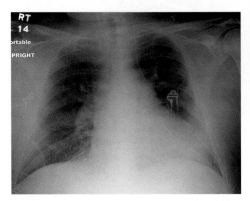

Figure 68.1

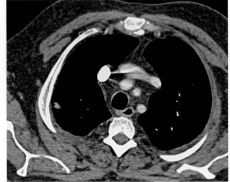

Figure 68.2

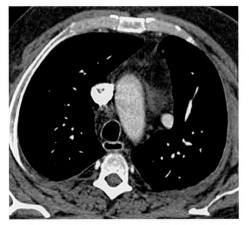

Figure 68.3

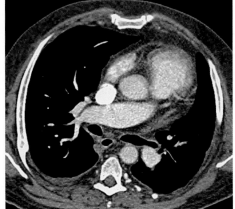

Figure 68.4

Case 68 Left Upper Lobe Partial Anomalous Pulmonary Venous Return (PAPVR)

Figure 68.5

Figure 68.6

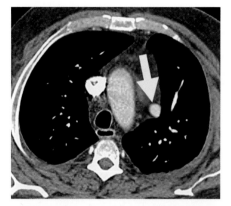

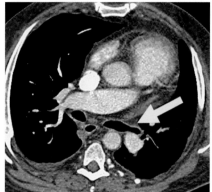

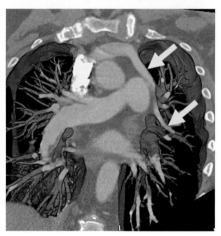

Figure 68.7

Findings

▶ Chest radiograph depicts a left internal jugular central line that courses laterally over the left upper lobe. Surrounding lucency in keeping with mediastinal fat is also noted.
▶ CT demonstrates a vertical vein (white arrow in Fig. 68.5) in the left para-aortic region.
▶ The left upper lobe pulmonary vein is not present in its normal location anterior to the left mainstem bronchus. White arrow in Figure 68.6 demarcates the expected location of the left superior pulmonary vein.
▶ Volume-rendered image shows the vertical vein in its entirety (arrows in Fig. 68.7).

Differential Diagnosis

▶ Based on the radiograph, the differential diagnosis for the catheter location would be in a left superior vena cava (SVC), left upper lobe anomalous pulmonary vein, left internal mammary vein, and extravascular. The ability to withdraw blood easily and the prior CT allow for the definitive diagnosis of left upper lobe PAPVR.

Teaching Points

▶ Left SVC and left superior PAPVR communicate with the left brachiocephalic vein.

▶ Left SVC drains into the coronary sinus and does not constitute a shunt. The course of a left SVC tends to be vertical.

▶ Left superior PAPVR takes a slightly more oblique course as it drains the left upper lobe into the left brachiocephalic vein. Left PAPVR is a left-to-right shunt.

▶ Of all the PAPVRs, left upper is the most common to be an isolated finding. Unlike right upper PAPVR, it is not usually seen with an atrial septal defect.

Management

▶ Usually left PAPVR is an incidental finding. When the shunt is large and symptomatic, surgery may be considered.

Further Reading

Ho ML, Bhalla S, Bierhals A, Gutierrez F. MDCT of partial anomalous pulmonary venous return (PAPVR) in adults. *J Thorac Imaging*. 2009 May;24(2):89-95.

Martinez-Jimenez S, Heyneman LE, McAdams HP, et al. Nonsurgical extracardiac vascular shunts in the thorax: clinical and imaging characteristics. *Radiographics*. 2010 Sep;30(5):e41.

History

▸ 35-year-old man with uncontrolled hypertension undergoes imaging.

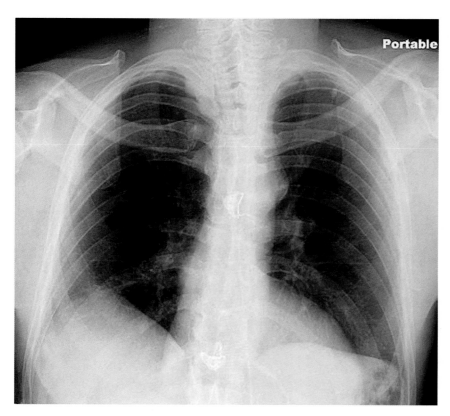

Figure 69.1

Case 69   Aortic Coarctation

Figure 69.2

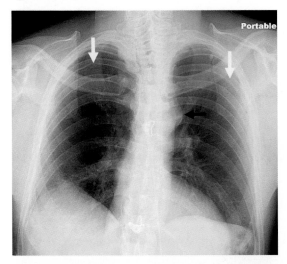

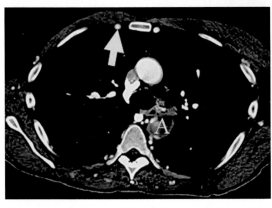

Figure 69.3

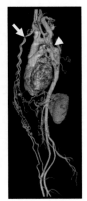

Figure 69.4

Findings

▸ Frontal radiograph shows bulging of the proximal descending aorta (black arrow in Fig. 69.2) from poststenotic dilation. The net effect is a "3 configuration" of the aorta.

▸ Inferior rib notching is present from collateral intercostal vessels (white arrows in Fig. 69.2). The enlarged intercostal vessels also present as a right paratracheal soft tissue mass.

▸ CT confirms the aortic narrowing (A = nearly obliterated descending aorta in Fig. 69.3; arrowhead = coarctation in Fig. 69.4). Note the enlarged internal mammary collaterals (arrows in Figs. 69.3 and 69.4), which reflect a pressure gradient across the stenosis.

Differential Diagnosis

▸ The main differential diagnosis for bilateral inferior rib notching consists of aortic coarctation and neurofibromatosis. Both may result in abnormal mediastinal contours. When the rib notching is unilateral, alternative diagnoses, such as ipsilateral Blalock-Taussig shunt, ipsilateral pulmonary artery aplasia, or atypical coarctation, should be considered.

Teaching Points

▶ Coarctation has an increased incidence in patients with Turner's syndrome and may be seen in association with intracardiac anomalies.

▶ Most often, aortic coarctation is seen as an isolated anomaly or in association with a bicuspid aortic valve. The area of narrowing usually involves the isthmus just distal to the left subclavian artery.

▶ Pseudocoarctation can occasionally mimic coarctation. In pseudocoarctation, a relative area of narrowing of the isthmus may be seen but no significant gradient exists. Collateral vessels are, therefore, absent. Pseudocoarctation may also result in a "3 configuration" of the aorta.

▶ Intercostal arteries, which allow for anastomoses between the internal mammary arteries and the descending aorta (ribs 3–8), may enlarge as these vessels bypass the coarctation.

▶ Both CT and MRI can be used to evaluate a suspected coarctation. An advantage of MR is the ability to estimate a gradient across the stenosis.

Management

▶ Previously aortic coarctation was managed operatively, but currently most coarctations are managed with endoluminal treatments—usually angioplasty followed by aortic stent placement.

Further Reading

Lee EY, Siegel MJ, Hildebolt CF, et al. MDCT evaluation of thoracic aortic anomalies in pediatric patients and young adults: comparison of axial, multiplanar, and 3D images. *AJR Am J Roentgenol.* 2004;182:777-784.

Maldonado JA, Henry T, Gutiérrez FR. Congenital thoracic vascular anomalies. *Radiol Clin North Am.* 2010 Jan;48(1):85-115.

History

▶ 54-year-old man with a history of sarcoidosis presents with massive hemoptysis.

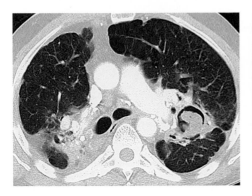

Figure 70.1

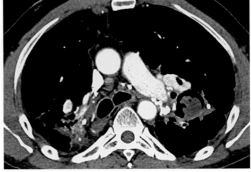

Figure 70.2

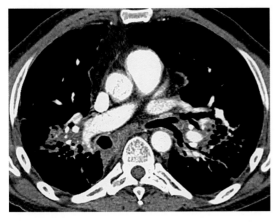

Figure 70.3

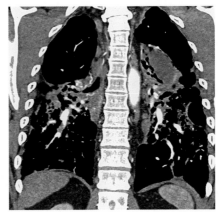

Figure 70.4

Case 70 Hemoptysis from Enlarged Bronchial Arteries

Figure 70.5

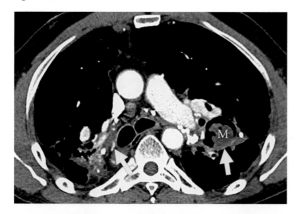

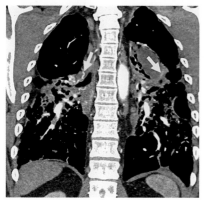

Figure 70.6

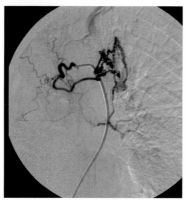

Figure 70.7

Findings

▶ CT shows upper lobe architectural changes with calcified mediastinal lymph nodes in keeping with sarcoidosis. A mycetoma (M in Fig. 70.5) is seen with enlarged bronchial arteries (arrows in Figs. 70.5 and 70.6), which are often easier to see on coronal images.

▶ Bronchial artery angiogram (Fig. 70.7) confirms the hypertrophied and irregular bronchial arteries.

Differential Diagnosis

▶ Differential diagnosis for hemoptysis includes enlarged bronchial arteries (in bronchiectasis, mycetomas, fibrosing mediastinitis, Eisenmenger's syndrome), pulmonary artery abnormalities (pseudoaneurysms), aortic bronchial fistulae, systemic feeding vessels, or endobronchial masses. In this case, the visualization of enlarged bronchial arteries makes bronchial artery etiology the most likely.

Teaching Points

▶ Hemoptysis can be life-threatening. When hemoptysis exceeds 300 to 600 mL in 24 hours, it is referred to as "massive hemoptysis." About 400 mL of blood is sufficient to result in asphyxiation.

▶ CTA can simultaneously assess the lungs, airways, pulmonary arteries, and bronchial arteries.

▶ The majority of bronchial arteries arise from the descending aorta at T5-T6.

▶ The most common bronchial artery pattern (seen in 40% of patients) consists of one right intercostobronchial trunk and two left bronchial arteries.

- Bronchial arteries outside of T5-T6 are *ectopic*. They may arise from the aortic arch, internal mammary arteries, thyrocervical trunk, subclavian artery, or inferior phrenic artery.
- Bronchiectasis or segmental pulmonary artery occlusion results in enlarged bronchial arteries and may present with hemoptysis. In congenital heart disease, these enlarged bronchial arteries are often referred to as major aortopulmonary collateral arteries (MAPCAS).
- Cavitary lesions, from old tuberculosis or mycetomas, may have fragile bronchial artery investment.

Management
- Bronchial artery embolization may stabilize a patient with life-threatening hemoptysis. Treatment is performed with medium-sized particles such as Gelfoam or polyvinyl alcohol (PVA). Coils are avoided because the larger size tends to occlude vessels too proximally and may prevent further angiographic intervention.
- When bronchial arteries are enlarged, patients tend to rebleed after embolization, especially when the underlying process is left untreated.

Further Reading
Yoon W, Kim JK, Kim YH, et al. Bronchial and nonbronchial systemic artery embolization for life-threatening hemoptysis: a comprehensive review. *Radiographics*. 2002 Nov-Dec;22(6):1395-1409.

History

▶ 15-year-old girl with history of repaired congenital heart disease presenting with progressive hypoxia.

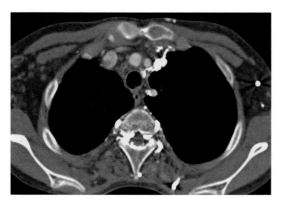

Figure 71.1

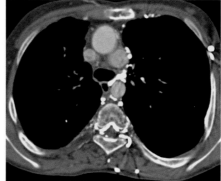

Figure 71.2

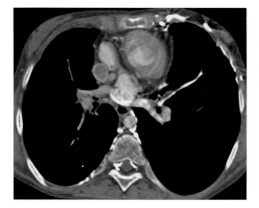

Figure 71.3

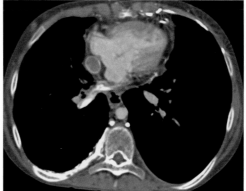

Figure 71.4

Case 71 Systemic-to-Left Atrial Collateral Vessels

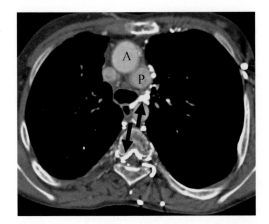

Figure 71.5

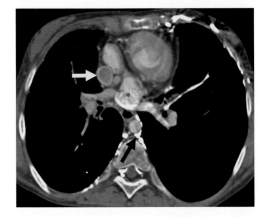

Figure 71.6

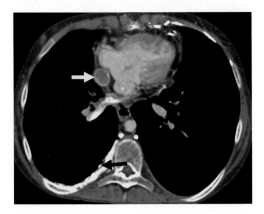

Figure 71.7

Findings

► CT images show D-transposition of the great vessels with the aorta (A) lying to the right and anterior to the pulmonary artery (P) and a univentricular heart. This was repaired with a total cavopulmonary shunt (white arrows in Figs. 71.6–71.7). The lack of opacification of the shunt is due to the phase of contrast, not thrombus.

► With injection of contrast into the left upper extremity, there is filling of numerous venous collaterals (black arrows in Figs. 71.5–71.7), including mediastinal and paravertebral venous plexuses. There is collateral contrast flow from systemic venous collaterals directly into the left atrium (black asterisk in Fig. 71.6) and into the left atrium via transpulmonary venous collateral flow These paths constitute right (unoxygenated systemic venous blood) to left (oxygenated systemic arterial blood) shunts.

Differential Diagnosis

► The differential diagnosis for visualization of multiple venous collaterals includes superior vena cava or brachiocephalic occlusion/stenosis with collaterals to other veins or venous collaterals with right-to-left shunts (which can be seen with or without central obstruction).

Teaching Points

► Collateral venous flow from the systemic venous system into the left atrium or pulmonary veins leads to a right-to-left shunt and may result in progressive hypoxia.

► These veno–veno collaterals are often seen as a complication of surgery for congenital heart disease (CHD), including Glenn, Fontan, and cavopulmonary shunts.

► Pulmonary arteriovenous malformations are another cause of hypoxia in the patient with a history of surgery for CHD. These can emulate those seen in hereditary hemorrhagic telangiectasia (see case 22).

► Veno–veno collaterals with right-to-left shunting can also be seen in the absence of CHD. These may follow superior vena caval or brachiocephalic vein occlusion.

► When collateral vessels are seen on CT, they should be followed to confirm that these shunts are absent.

Management

► Endovascular embolization of these collateral venous channels is now the treatment of choice, especially in the CHD patient.

► At the time of the staged surgical procedure for correcting univentricular conditions, any collateral channels to the left atrium are ligated.

Further Reading

Andrews RE, Tulloh RM, Anderson DR. Coil occlusion of systemic venous collaterals in hypoplastic left heart syndrome. *Heart*. 2002 Aug;88(2):167-169.

Bardo DM, Frankel DG, Applegate KE, et al. Hypoplastic left heart syndrome. *Radiographics*. May 2001;21:705-717.

History

► 53-year-old woman presents with shortness of breath and arm swelling.

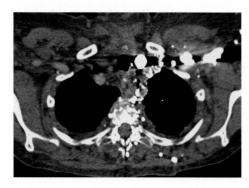

Figure 72.1

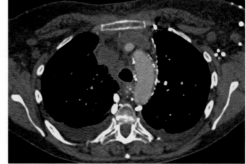

Figure 72.2

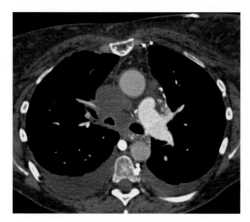

Figure 72.3

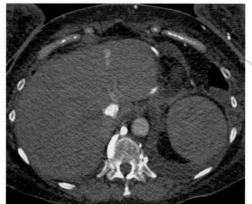

Figure 72.4

Case 72 Superior Vena Cava Syndrome/Obstruction (Secondary to Non-Small Cell Lung Carcinoma)

Figure 72.5

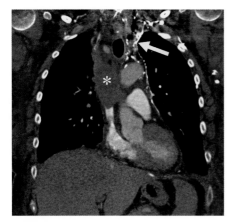

Figure 72.6

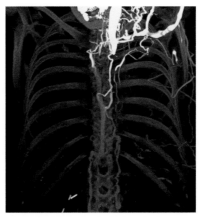

Findings

▶ With injection from the left upper extremity, dense contrast flows in numerous collateral veins (arrow in Fig. 72.5). Dense enhancement in the anterior aspect of the left hepatic lobe is known as the hot quadrate sign (Fig. 72.4).

▶ Right paratracheal/hilar soft tissue mass (asterisk in Fig. 72.5) obstructs the superior vena cava.

Differential Diagnosis

▶ When multiple collateral veins are present on power injection and altered collateral paths are seen, the first consideration is the level of the obstruction (subclavian vein, brachiocephalic vein, or superior vena cava [SVC]). Once the level is found, the cause can easily be deciphered.

Teaching Points

▶ SVC obstruction is most commonly due to neoplasm, usually lung cancer, fibrosing mediastinitis, indwelling venous catheter, or pacemaker. SVC occlusion can result from direct invasion or external compression.

▶ SVC syndrome may present with neck and upper extremity swelling.

▶ CT is useful in determining the cause (malignant vs. benign), and the presence or absence of thrombus. Acute thrombosis will expand the SVC. In chronic occlusion, the SVC becomes diminutive and difficult to visualize.

▶ CT in a slightly delayed phase (60–90 seconds) is useful to assess for thrombus and SVC patency.

▶ Numerous collateral venous pathways can be recruited in the setting of SVC occlusion. If the occlusion is below the azygos arch, dense contrast enhancement of the azygos system is seen with retrograde flow via collaterals to the inferior vena cava. If the occlusion is above the azygos arch, the azygos system can serve as an antegrade path for blood return to the right heart.

▶ Contrast enhancement in the anterior margin of the liver adjacent to the gallbladder fossa and porta hepatis, frequently referred to as the hot quadrate lobe, is due to collateral circulation from epigastric veins to the left portal vein.

Management

▶ Transvenous venoplasty and stenting can be used for treatment. In cases of obstruction due to malignant invasion, stents can be used to bypass the affected region.

Further Reading

Sheth S, Ebert MD, Fishman EK. Superior vena cava obstruction evaluation with MDCT. *AJR Am J Roentgenol.* 2010 Apr;194(4):W336-46.

Part 9   Thoracic Outlet Cases

History

▶ 19-year-old college baseball pitcher with right arm pain and swelling undergoes MR angiography.

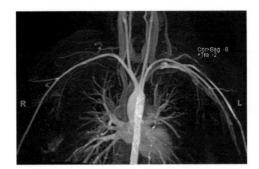

Figure 73.1

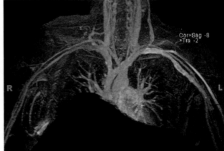

Figure 73.2

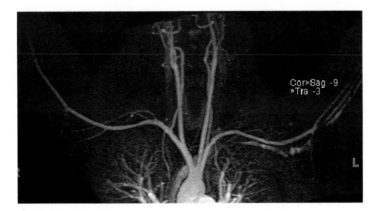

Figure 73.3

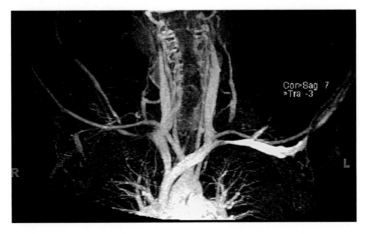

Figure 73.4

Case 73 Thoracic Outlet Syndrome

Figure 73.5

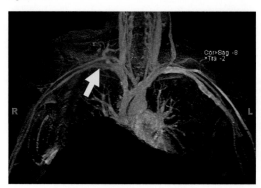

Figure 73.6

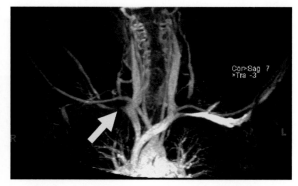

Findings

► MRA for thoracic outlet syndrome is performed with arms down (adduction) (Figs. 73.1 and 73.2) and arms up (abduction) (Figs. 73.3 and 73.4). Both arterial and venous phases are shown.

► Arterial-phase images (Figs. 73.1 and 73.3) show no significant narrowing of the subclavian artery in either position.

► Venous-phase images show near-complete occlusion of the right subclavian vein (arrows in Figs. 73.5 and 73.6) with arms up.

Differential Diagnosis

► The differential diagnosis of apparent narrowing in this location includes thoracic outlet syndrome or artifact from pooling of gadolinium in the vein. For this reason, the arm contralateral to the suspected side (in this case the left arm) is selected for injection.

Teaching Points

► The diagnosis of thoracic outlet syndrome with imaging requires dynamic maneuvers to bring out the stenosis. Care must be taken to avoid overlooking this condition by relying on adduction (arms down) angiography alone.

► The area of narrowing is usually between the first rib or a cervical rib and the clavicle.
  The narrowing may be related to the bone, the anterior scalene muscle, or a fibrous band.

► Imaging must also evaluate for thrombus in the artery or vein that may serve as a source for embolism. If this were the case, anticoagulation would be necessary prior to any definitive treatment.

► Occasionally, an aneurysm of the subclavian artery may be a manifestation of thoracic outlet syndrome. The aneurysm is believed to result from repetitive microtrauma.

► Venous thrombosis is the setting of thoracic outlet syndrome is sometimes referred to as *effort thrombosis* or *Paget-Schroetter syndrome.*

► MRA cannot exclude neurogenic thoracic outlet syndrome.

Management

► Depending on the clinical scenario, this may be treated with conservative management such as stretching, steroids, and anticoagulation.

► In certain situations, surgical decompression or angioplasty may be required.

Further Reading

Demondion X, Herbinet P, Van Sint Jan S, et al. Imaging assessment of thoracic outlet syndrome. *Radiographics.* 2006 Nov-Dec;26(6): 1735-1750.

Sanders RJ, Hammond SL, Rao NM. Diagnosis of thoracic outlet syndrome. *J Vasc Surg.* 2007 Sep;46(3):601-604.

History

▶ 44-year-old woman presents with a tender, palpable mass.

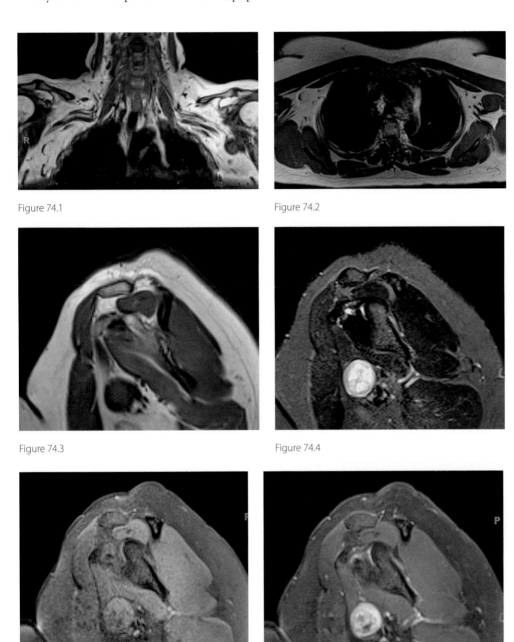

Figure 74.1

Figure 74.2

Figure 74.3

Figure 74.4

Figure 74.5

Figure 74.6

Case 74 Brachial Plexus Mass (Left Axillary Schwannoma Arising from Lateral Cord of the Brachial Plexus and the Musculocutaneous Nerve)

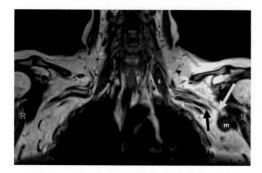

Figure 74.7

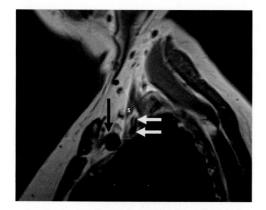

Figure 74.8

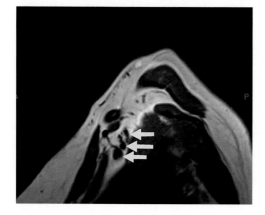

Figure 74.9

Findings

▶ T1-weighted MR shows a mass from the lateral cord/musculocutaneous nerve of the brachial plexus (Fig. 74.7; white arrow = brachial plexus; black arrow = subclavian artery; m = mass and s = anterior scalene muscle).

▶ The mass is isointense to muscle on the sagittal T1-weighted image (Fig. 74.3) and hyperintense on sagittal T2/STIR (Fig. 74.4). The mass has a targetoid enhancement pattern with gadolinium (Fig. 74.6).

Differential Diagnosis

▶ Differential diagnosis for the mass would include lymphadenopathy or nerve sheath tumor (schwannoma). Once the connection to the brachial plexus and the enhancement pattern is seen, schwannoma is favored.

Teaching Points

▶ The brachial plexus provides sensory and motor innervation to the upper extremities and is formed by the ventral rami of spinal nerves C5–T1.

▶ The ventral rami join to form three trunks, which give rise to three anterior divisions and three posterior divisions. These divisions eventually merge to form three cords, which end in the terminal branches (nerves).

▶ The subclavian artery can be useful in finding the brachial plexus as the plexus always travels slightly superior to the artery (Fig. 74.8 [s = anterior scalene; top white arrow = brachial plexus; inferior white arrow = subclavian artery; vertical black arrow = brachiocephalic vein] and Fig. 74.9 [superior arrow = brachial plexus; middle arrow = subclavian artery; inferior arrow = subclavian vein].

▶ MR is the preferred method for imaging the plexus.

▶ Tumors of the brachial plexus are usually neurogenic (neurofibromas, schwannomas, malignant nerve sheath tumors).

▶ 20% of all peripheral nerve sheath tumors arise in the brachial plexus. Neurofibromas are the most common, followed by schwannomas. Malignant nerve sheath tumors are rare and are usually seen with neurofibromatosis.

▶ Non-neurogenic tumors include desmoids and lipomas.

▶ Lung cancers and metastatic lymphadenopathy may involve the brachial plexus. True hematogenous metastases to the plexus are rare.

Management

▶ Although benign, schwannomas of the plexus may be resected because of pain.

Further Reading

Todd M, Shah GV, Mukherji SK. MR imaging of brachial plexus. *Top Magn Reson Imaging.* 2004 Apr;15(2):113-125.

History

▶ 44-year-old man presents with fever and productive cough with blood-tinged sputum for over 2 weeks.

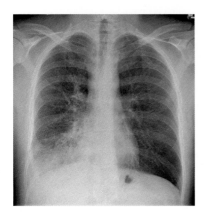

Figure 75.1

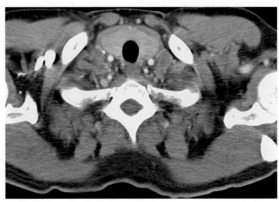

Figure 75.2a

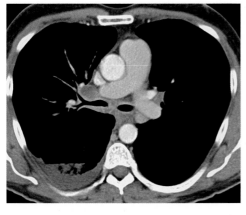

Figure 75.2b

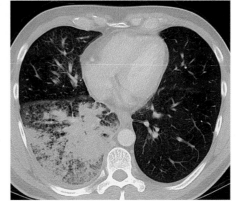

Figure 75.2c

Case 75   Supraclavicular Lymphadenopathy (from Metastatic Non-Small Lung Cancer)

Figure 75.3

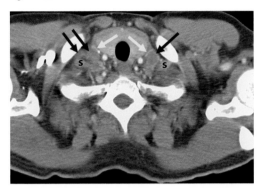

Figure 75.4

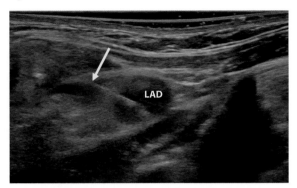

Findings

▶ Chest radiograph (Fig. 75.1) shows right lower lobe airspace disease with a small effusion and a large right hilum. This was originally thought to represent pneumonia.

▶ CT (Fig. 75.2) performed after failure of improvement in symptoms with 10 days of antibiotics shows a spiculated mass in the center with associated right, subcarinal, and left hilar low-attenuating lymphadenopathy. Image through the thoracic inlet shows bilateral supraclavicular lymphadenopathy (Fig. 75.3; white arrows = compressed internal jugular veins; s = anterior scalene muscles; black arrows = lymphadenopathy).

Differential Diagnosis

▶ For the thoracic outlet findings, the differential diagnosis includes lymphadenopathy or rarely (in the setting of neurofibromatosis) multiple nerve sheath tumors. The persistent consolidation despite antibiotic treatment would prompt consideration of a resistant infection, inflammatory pneumonia (such as organizing pneumonia), or neoplasm. Given the supraclavicular lymphadenopathy, neoplasm would be favored.

Teaching Points

▶ CT is frequently used to diagnose and stage lung cancer. Supraclavicular nodes (or lymph nodes above the level of the left brachiocephalic vein) can be hard to detect.

▶ The key to detection is to first identify the anterior scalene muscles. Any extra mass that resembles the muscle is probably a lymph node.

▶ Lymph nodes >7 mm are considered enlarged.

▶ <50% of pathologically enlarged lymph nodes will be detected by palpation, making imaging important in the diagnosis of supraclavicular lymphadenopathy.

▶ The presence of metastases in supraclavicular lymph nodes in lung cancer is critical in non-small cell lung cancer because it defines the N status as N3, which makes the stage at least IIIB (inoperable).

Management

▶ Diagnosing supraclavicular lymphadenopathy allows for the least invasive method to diagnose a pulmonary or mediastinal process. Percutaneous ultrasound biopsy can be used quite effectively, as it was in this case (Fig. 75.4 [arrow = needle, LAD = lymphadenopathy]).

Further Reading

van Overhagen H, Brakel K, Heijenbrok MW, et al. Metastases in supraclavicular lymph nodes in lung cancer: assessment with palpation, US, and CT. *Radiology*. 2004 Jul;232(1):75-80.

History

► 55-year-old woman with newly diagnosed hypercalcemia and hyperparathyroidism.

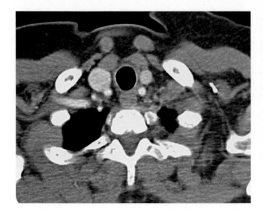

Figure 76.1a

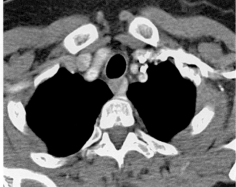

Figure 76.1b

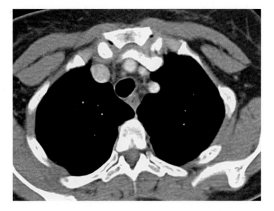

Figure 76.1c

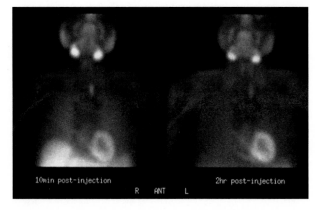

Figure 76.2

Case 76   Ectopic Parathyroid Adenoma

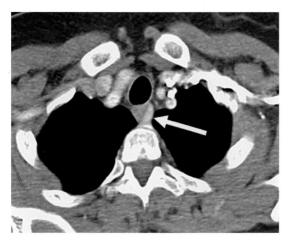

Figure 76.3

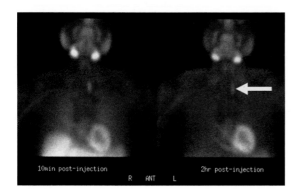

Figure 76.4

Findings

▶ CT images are deceptively normal at first glance but on closer inspection show a hypervascular nodule adjacent to the esophagus (arrow in Fig. 76.3)

▶ The nature of the nodule is confirmed on Tc99m-sestamibi parathyroid scintigraphy, which shows that the nodule has persistent uptake on the 2-hour image (arrow in Fig. 76.4).

Differential Diagnosis

▶ For the hypervascular nodule on CT at the level of the thoracic outlet, the differential includes a hypervascular lymph node, parathyroid adenoma, mediastinal paraganglioma, or vascular lesion (aneurysm or varix).

Teaching Points

▶ Primary hyperparathyroidism is a common endocrine disorder, affecting approximately 1 in 500 women and 1 in 2,000 men. In >90% of cases surgical removal of the four parathyroid glands is curative.

▶ Normally, the parathyroid glands are not seen on CT.

▶ Ectopic adenomas have been reported in 20% to 25% of cases of primary hyperparathyroidism.

▶ Most ectopic adenomas are between the hyoid bone and the tracheal carina.

- In the thoracic outlet, the adenomas tend to be posteriorly located in the retropharyngeal or retrovisceral spaces, although they may be adjacent to the carotid space.
- In the upper mediastinum, adenomas are typically in the anterior mediastinum. They may be confused with residual thymic tissue.
- On CT, adenomas tend to be homogeneous and a majority (>85%) are hyperenhancing (compared to muscle).
- Because a majority of ectopic parathyroid adenomas tend to be around 1 cm, detection relies on an understanding of the complex anatomy of the thoracic outlet.

Management

- Surgical removal of the hyperfunctioning parathyroid gland is the primary curative treatment.
- Over the past decade minimally invasive parathyroidectomy has become the preferred surgical approach. Success relies on accurate preoperative localization of the parathyroid lesions.
- Ultrasound and Tc-99m sestamibi scintigraphy, particularly when complemented by single photon emission computed tomography (SPECT), are currently the imaging techniques of choice for preoperative localization of parathyroid adenomas; a combination of the two methods further improves the sensitivity and accuracy of detection.
- CT is less commonly used for preoperative localization and is usually reserved for cases of failed parathyroidectomy, for the detection of suspected ectopic glands. SPECT/CT appears promising, but further studies are needed to evaluate its role.

Further Reading

Randall GJ, Zald PB, Cohen JI, Hamilton BE. Contrast-enhanced MDCT characteristics of parathyroid adenomas. *AJR Am J Roentgenol*. 2009;193(2):W139-143.

Part 10

Diaphragmatic Conditions

History

▶ 54-year-old woman is imaged for worsening shortness of breath.

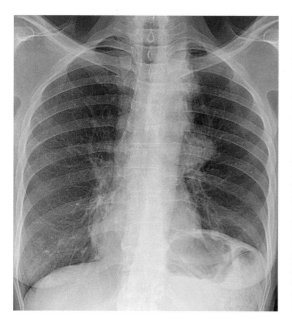

Figure 77.1

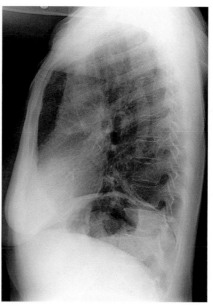

Figure 77.2

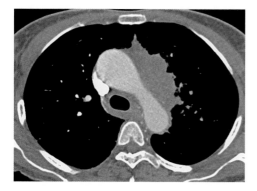

Figure 77.3

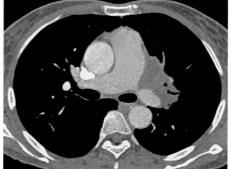

Figure 77.4

Case 77 Phrenic Nerve Invasion with Left Hemidiaphragm Paralysis (from Non-Small Cell Lung Cancer)

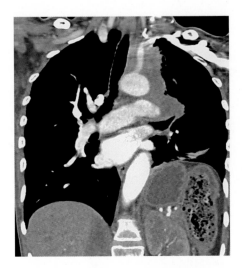

Figure 77.5

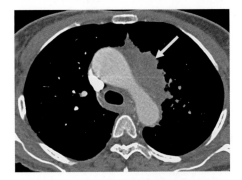

Figure 77.6

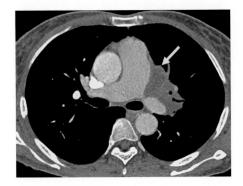

Figure 77.7

Findings

▶ Two-view chest radiograph (Figs. 77.1 and 77.2) shows massive mediastinal and left hilar lymphadenopathy. The left hemidiaphragm is also elevated.

▶ CT images (Figs. 77.3 and 77.4) confirm the massive lymphadenopathy but do not show any parenchymal nodules. Elevated left hemidiaphragm is more easily appreciated on the coronal reconstruction (Fig. 77.5).

Differential Diagnosis

▶ Although the lymphadenopathy has a wide differential diagnosis, the elevated hemidiaphragm does not. The main differential consists of elevated hemidiaphragm from malignant phrenic nerve invasion versus prior phrenic nerve injury. The shape of the hemidiaphragm would not support a hernia or eventration.

Teaching Points

▶ The phrenic nerves are only rarely seen on routine CT.

▶ The phrenic nerves run along the lateral mediastinum. The right phrenic nerve usually runs lateral to the right brachiocephalic vein and the superior vena cava. The left phrenic nerve passes along the lateral aspect of the aortic arch (arrows in Figs. 77.6 and 77.7 show expected location of the left phrenic nerve).

▶ The phrenic nerves subsequently pass anterior to their respective pulmonary hila and then inferiorly along the pericardial surfaces.

▶ Phrenic nerve compromise can present with diaphragmatic paralysis with elevation or persistent hiccups.

▶ Primary tumors of the phrenic nerves are rare but can be seen in neurofibromatosis. Metastatic disease involvement from primary lung cancer is more common.

▶ Injury to the phrenic nerves can occur from penetrating injury, surgery, and trauma.

Management

▶ The presence of phrenic nerve invasion affects the T status of lung cancer staging, making the lesion at least T3 inv (invasion or central). Other defining criteria for the T3 inv group include direct invasion of the chest wall, diaphragm, mediastinal pleura, or parietal pericardium.

▶ If there is doubt of the phrenic nerve invasion, confirmation with fluoroscopy, inspiration/expiration CT, or MR may be performed.

Further Reading

Aquino SL, Duncan GR, Hayman LA. Nerves of the thorax: atlas of normal and pathologic findings. *Radiographics*. 2001; Sep-Oct; 21(5):1275-1281.

Detterbeck FC, Boffa DJ, Tanoue LT. The new lung cancer staging system. *Chest*. 2009 Jul;136(1):260-271.

History

▶ 61-year-old woman with a history of lung cancer presents with severe dyspnea.

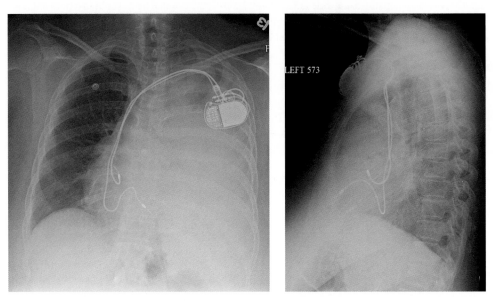

Figure 78.1   Figure 78.2

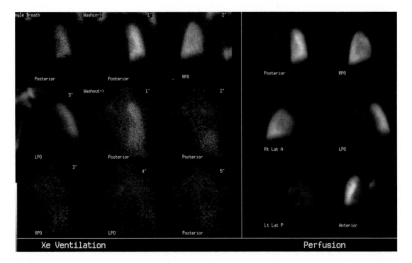

Figure 78.3

Case 78 Inverted Hemidiaphragm from Malignant Effusion

Figure 78.4

Figure 78.5

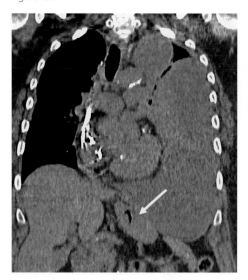

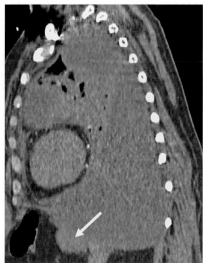

Findings

▶ Two-view chest radiograph shows near-complete opacification of the left hemothorax with mass effect on the heart and mediastinum (Figs. 78.1 and 78.2). The images also show anterior and inferior displacement of the stomach (arrow in Figs. 78.4 and 78.5).

▶ Ventilation-perfusion scintigraphy (Fig. 78.3) was performed to evaluate the acute onset of dyspnea. Note the left lung has very little perfusion or ventilation, owing to the effects of the large effusion under tension and the central mass.

Differential Diagnosis

▶ Inverted diaphragm from a large pleural effusion (as in Case 3) heads the differential diagnosis from malignancy, hemothorax, empyema, or chylothorax.

Teaching Points

▶ One unusual complication of a large pleural effusion is inversion of the ipsilateral hemidiaphragm.

▶ The consequence of the large effusion is that now the two hemidiaphragms will move in opposite directions during respiration. This may result in gas going from one lung to the other (so-called pendelluft or pendulum respiration).

▶ The increased dead space, in addition to the tension on the pulmonary vascularity, can result in profound dyspnea.

▶ Chest radiograph findings of inversion rely on displacement of the stomach (compare arrow in Fig. 78.6 and arrow on a subsequent radiograph in
Fig. 78.7) inferiorly and the splenic flexure (c in Figs. 78.6 and 78.7). On a lateral projection, both will be displaced anteriorly. For this reason, inversion is better seen on the left.

▶ On CT and ultrasound, inverted hemidiaphragm may be confusing on images through the upper abdomen as the relationship of the pleural effusion and the peritoneal space is altered. The pleural effusion will now be central to the peritoneal contents.

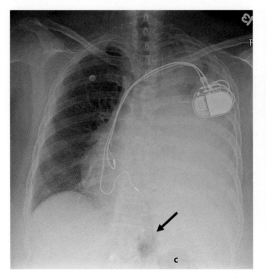

Figure 78.6

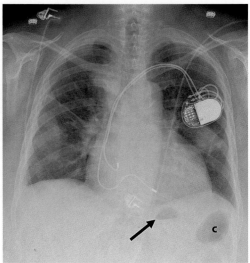

Figure 78.7

Management

▶ Effusions with inversion of the hemidiaphragm require drainage on an urgent/emergent basis. Note how the stomach (arrow in Fig. 78.7) and colon (c in Fig. 78.7) return to a more normal location on the radiograph obtained 2 months after the effusion was drained and patient underwent pleurodesis.

Further Reading

Wang JS, Tseng CH. Changes in pulmonary mechanics and gas exchange after thoracentesis on patients with inversion of a hemidiaphragm secondary to large pleural effusion. *Chest.* 1995;107(6):1610-1614.

History

▶ 35-year-old man presents with shortness of breath 4 months after falling out of a tree.

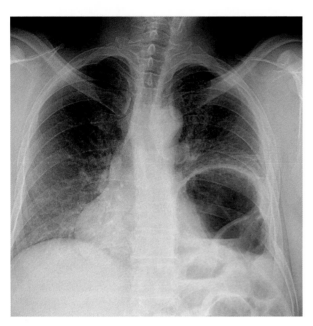

Figure 79.1

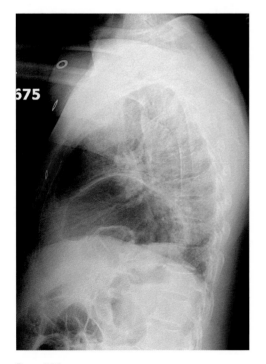

Figure 79.2

Case 79   Ruptured Diaphragm

Figure 79.3

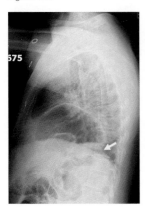

Figure 79.4

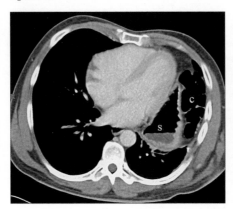

Figure 79.5

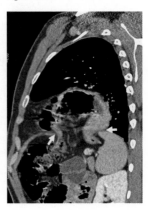

Findings

▶ Chest radiograph demonstrates elevation of the gastric bubble. The contour of the apparent diaphragm is irregular and the heart is shifted rightward.

▶ Lateral examination demonstrates a focal extrusion of the stomach above the level of the left hemidiaphragm with a neck (arrow in Fig. 79.3).

▶ CT images demonstrate stomach (s in Fig. 79.4) and colon (c in Fig. 79.4) abutting the chest wall.

▶ Sagittal reconstruction demonstrates a large diaphragmatic defect (white arrows in Fig. 79.5) with herniation of the stomach, colon, and mesenteric vessels/fat into the thoracic cavity. There is a waist at the level of the herniation (*collar sign*).

Differential Diagnosis

▶ Differential diagnosis for apparent elevation of the left hemidiaphragm consists of traumatic rupture, paralysis, or eventration. Shift of the heart rightward and the normal posterior sulcus would argue against paralysis. The acute angle between the stomach and left hemidiaphragm (posterior arrow in Fig. 79.4) would favor traumatic rupture over eventration.

Teaching Points

▶ Traumatic rupture of the diaphragm is seen in <5% of blunt trauma cases and is harder to image in penetrating trauma.

▶ Elevated abdominal pressures force abdominal organs into the pleural space. Positive-pressure ventilation may mask rupture by reducing the pleural pressure gradient and preventing herniation.

▶ Left-sided injuries are easier to identify on imaging.

▶ Elevated diaphragm in the setting of trauma should raise the suspicion of a diaphragmatic hernia.

▶ Chest radiograph findings include apparent diaphragmatic elevation, irregular or discontinuous diaphragmatic contour, abnormal course of a feeding tube, or gas-containing viscera above the diaphragm.

▶ MDCT findings include the collar sign, the dependent viscera sign (stomach resting on the posterior chest wall), herniated viscus or mesentery, large defect in the diaphragm, retraction of the injured part of the muscle adjacent to the tear, and the *cottage bread sign* (referring to a right injury with herniated liver simulating brioche).

Management

▶ A diaphragmatic herniation requires prompt surgical attention due to the increased risk of strangulation of the herniated viscera.

Further Reading

Iochum S, Ludig T, Walter T, et al. Imaging of diaphragmatic injury: a diagnostic challenge? *Radiographics*. 2002 Oct.;22:S103-S116.

Part 11 **Pulmonary Nodules and Masses**

History

▶ 75-year-old woman with a history of mastectomy for breast cancer presents with a solitary pulmonary nodule.

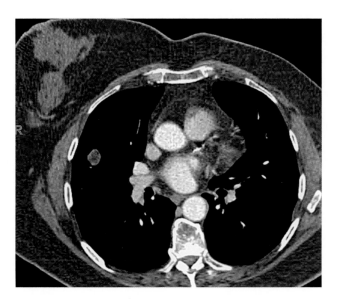

Figure 80.1

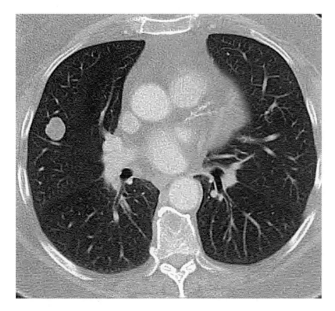

Figure 80.2

Case 80   Hamartoma

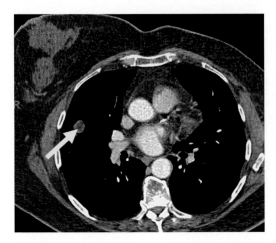

Figure 80.3

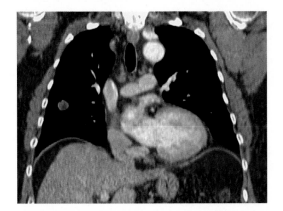

Figure 80.4

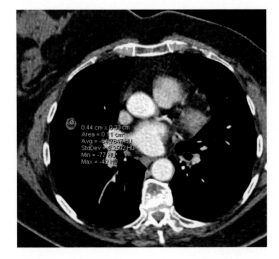

Figure 80.5

Findings

- ► CT images show a well-defined pulmonary nodule with central fat attenuation (arrow in Fig. 80.3). Multiplanar reconstruction (Fig. 80.3) confirms that the low attenuation is central in another plane and not simply volume averaging.
- ► HU measurement (Fig. 80.5) with the region of interest in the center shows the average HU = –64.7 (range –42 to –77 HU).

Differential Diagnosis

- ► The differential diagnosis for a solitary pulmonary nodule is extensive, but when fat attenuation is present, the list becomes quite short and consists of hamartoma or lipoid pneumonia. The borders of a hamartoma are smooth, and for this reason, hamartoma is the preferred diagnosis in this case.

Teaching Points

- ► Hamartomas account for 10% of all resected solitary pulmonary nodules and are among the more common benign pulmonary nodules.
- ► Popcorn calcification is typical of hamartomas and is due to chondroid calcification.
- ► Another pathognomonic feature of hamartomas is the presence of fat (with internal densities of –40 to –120 HU). In fact, the presence of fat allows for a confident diagnosis in a smooth nodule measuring <2.5 cm in diameter.
- ► At least one third of hamartomas do not contain fat or calcium.
- ► Hamartomas should not have increased uptake of FDG on PET. They may occasionally enhance on CT, especially in the regions of cartilaginous septa.
- ► Lipoid pneumonia can rarely present as a solitary pulmonary nodule. The border of an area of lipoid pneumonia will be spiculated. Lipoid pneumonia is more common in the dependent portions of the lungs.
- ► Care must be taken in observing the presence of fat within the nodule. Occasionally, the adjacent lung will volume average with a nodule and simulate fat. To avoid this pitfall, fat should be observed on more than one image or in more than one plane.

Management

- ► A hamartoma is a benign lesion. When CT pathognomonic features are present (namely fat), the workup can end.

Further Reading

Edey AJ, Hansell DM. Incidentally detected small pulmonary nodules on CT. *Clin Radiol.* 2009 Sep;64(9):872-884.
Gaerte SC, Meyer CA, Winer-Muram HT, et al. Fat-containing lesions of the chest. *Radiographics.* 2002 Oct;22 Spec No:S61-78.

History

▶ 78-year-old woman presents with shortness of breath.

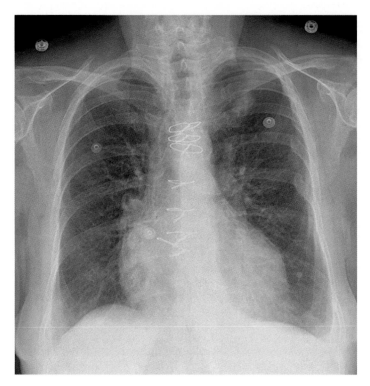

Figure 81.1

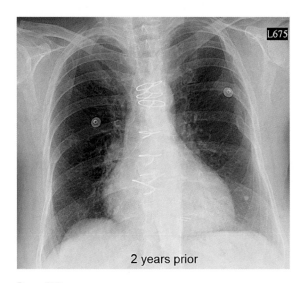

Figure 81.2

Case 81   Adenocarcinoma of Lung as a Solitary Pulmonary Nodule

Figure 81.3

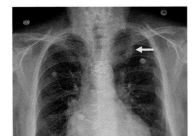

Figure 81.4

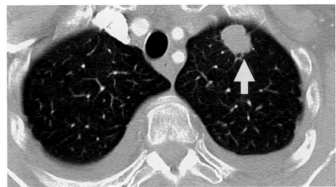

Findings

▶ Chest radiograph demonstrates asymmetric nodular density overlying the left first rib (arrow in Fig. 81.3) not seen on a prior radiograph (Fig. 81.2).

▶ CT confirms the 2.5-cm lobulated solitary, solid pulmonary nodule without any associated satellite lesion (arrow in Fig. 81.4).

Differential Diagnosis

▶ Differential diagnosis for a solitary pulmonary nodule (SPN) is extensive and based on the chest radiograph would include bronchogenic cancer, first rib calcification (or callus), benign lesion (including hamartoma or granuloma), or even a round pneumonia.

Teaching Points

▶ SPN is defined as an isolated lung lesion <3 cm without adenopathy or pleural involvement. When a lesion is >3 cm, it is referred to as a *mass*.

▶ Probability of malignancy is based on the patient's history. Risk factors include history of malignancy, smoking history, advanced age, exposure to radon or asbestos, pulmonary fibrosis, and family history.

▶ Although the literature reports 15% to 70% of SPNs will be malignant, 30% to 50% of lung adenocarcinomas will present as an SPN.

▶ Radiographic feature suggesting malignancy include doubling time >30 days but <400 days, size (>80% of SPNs >2 cm will be malignant), and lobulated or spiculated border. Of these, the growth rate is most concerning.

▶ Ground-glass nodules may have >400-day doubling times when they are bronchioloalveolar carcinoma.

▶ Benign calcification patterns include central calcification, lamellated (onion-skin), popcorn-like, and complete calcification. Eccentric calcification is not helpful.

▶ Satellite nodules, symptoms of pneumonia, long z-axis, or doubling time <30 days suggest that a lesion may be inflammatory or infectious.

Management

▶ A nodule of this size has a high likelihood of being cancer and may proceed to surgical resection. If the patient is not a surgical candidate, tissue sampling may be needed for radiation and chemotherapy.

▶ Occasionally PET may be used to detect occult metastases or to help determine the likelihood of malignancy of an SPN. In these situations a standardized uptake value of >2.5 may be used to suggest malignancy, keeping in mind that granulomas may also have high uptake.

Further Reading

Truong MT, Sabloff BS, Ko JP. Multidetector CT of solitary pulmonary nodules. *Radiol Clin North Am.* 2010 Jan;48(1):141-155.

History

► 55-year-old man who will serve a kidney donor for his brother receives a screening chest radiograph.

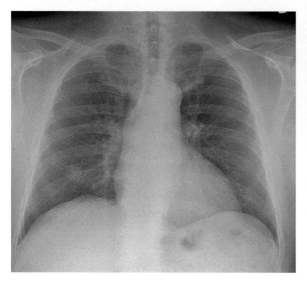

Figure 82.1

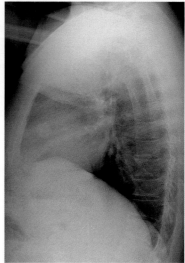

Figure 82.2

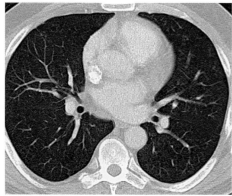

Figure 82.3

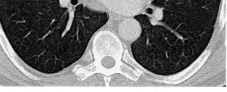

Figure 82.4

Case 82 Granuloma (from Histoplasmosis)

Figure 82.5

Figure 82.6

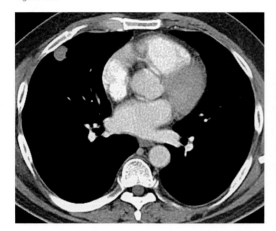
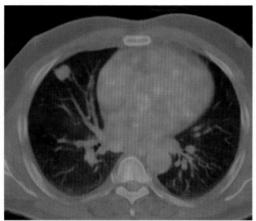

Findings

► Chest radiograph shows a well-defined right middle lobe nodule (Figs. 82.1 and 82.2).
► On CT (Figs. 82.3–82.5) the nodule is isoattenuating to muscle without visible fat or calcium. On lung windows, the nodule is fairly smooth-bordered. In Figure 82.3 tiny satellite nodules can be seen superiorly.
► On FDG-PET/CT (Fig. 82.6) the nodule does not demonstrate any increased FDG uptake. The standardized uptake value (SUV) is <1.5.

Differential Diagnosis

► Differential diagnosis for a solitary pulmonary nodule (SPN) is vast but in this case was headed by infectious granuloma, bronchogenic carcinoma, hamartoma, or carcinoid tumor. As the patient had no history of malignancy, metastases were felt to be unlikely.

Teaching Points

► Infectious granulomas may follow mycobacterial or fungal infection.
► Granulomas, especially from tuberculosis and histoplasmosis, often calcify. When the entire nodule is calcified in a solid or lamellated pattern, diagnosis can readily be made. Other patterns of calcification, such as eccentric, cannot be used to distinguish granulomas from malignancy.
► Granulomas tend to be well defined and round. Rarely, they may have surrounding fibrosis that can result in a spiculated border, simulating bronchogenic cancer.
► Small satellite nodules suggest that the dominant nodule is benign.
► PET can be used for the evaluation of an SPN but should be done in the context of the pretest likelihood of malignancy. Typically, an SUV <2.5 suggests a benign etiology. Semisolid or ground-glass nodules, however, can be malignant and have an SUV <2.5. Occasionally, a granuloma can be metabolically active with an SUV >2.5.

Management

► If a lesion is known to be a granuloma, because of a benign calcium pattern, it is left alone.
► In this case, the approach to the lesion was based on the clinical situation. Typically, the negative PET and low-pretest likelihood would have resulted in annual follow-up CT for 2 years. Because the patient wanted a definitive diagnosis so he could donate his kidney, a wedge resection was performed.

Further Reading
Truong MT, Sabloff BS, Ko JP. Multidetector CT of solitary pulmonary nodules. *Radiol Clin North Am.* 2010 Jan;48(1):141-155.

History

▶ 19-year-old girl with new-onset wheezing and hemoptysis. She has a history of right knee sarcoma resected 2 years ago.

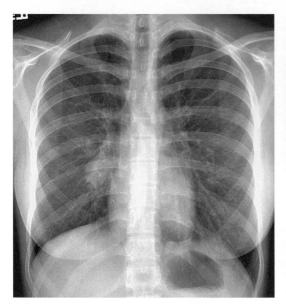

Figure 83.1

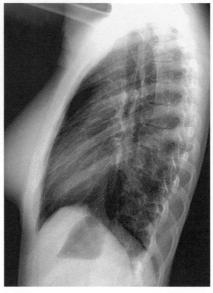

Figure 83.2

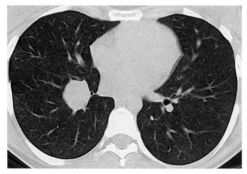

Figure 83.3

Figure 83.4

Case 83 Solitary Pulmonary Metastasis (from Osteosarcoma)

Figure 83.5

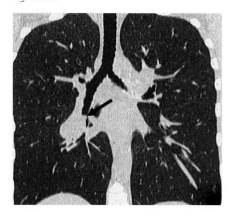

Findings

▸ Chest radiograph shows a right hilar nodule (Figs. 83.1 and 83.2) that was not present 3 months ago.

▸ On CT the nodule is isoattenuating to muscle without fat or calcium. On lung windows, the nodule is smooth and abuts the bronchus.

▸ CT reconstructions shows the endobronchial component (arrow in Fig. 83.5).

Differential Diagnosis

▸ The differential diagnosis for a solitary pulmonary nodule (SPN) is based on the patient's age and medical history. Metastasis is most likely, but somewhat unusual given the rapid growth and solitary nature. Other considerations include fungal infection, carcinoid tumor (unusual given rapid growth), and inflammatory myofibroblastic tumor. In an older patient, bronchogenic carcinoma might be considered.

Teaching Points

▸ Classically, metastases tend to be multiple and smoothly marginated. Their borders tend to be smoother than those of bronchogenic carcinoma.

▸ Location should not be used to assess the probability that a nodule is a metastasis.

▸ Metastases tend to be multiple but in about 10% of cases may present as a solitary nodule. A solitary metastasis tends to be less spiculated and smoother than a bronchogenic carcinoma. Solitary metastases may be seen with colon carcinoma, melanoma, renal cell carcinoma, testicular carcinoma, and sarcoma.

▸ Solitary metastasis is unusual in breast cancer, gastric cancer, cervical cancer, or head and neck cancers. When a solitary nodule or mass is encountered in patients with these cancers, consideration should be given to a primary lung cancer.

▸ Occasionally, metastases from sarcomas may calcify. These tend to demonstrate increased uptake on bone scintigraphy, a feature that may be useful in distinguishing them from granulomas.

▸ Besides presenting with calcification or as a solitary lesion, sarcoma metastases may grow rapidly. They may also present with a pneumothorax.

Management

▸ Management depends on the primary tumor.

▸ Because sarcomas respond so poorly to chemotherapy and radiotherapy, treatment is surgical. In this case a lower lobe resection was performed.

Further Reading

Quint LE, Park CH, Iannettoni MD. Solitary pulmonary nodules in patients with extrapulmonary neoplasms. *Radiology*. 2000 Oct;217(1):257-261.

History

▶ 50-year-old woman with hemoptysis and increasing shortness of breath undergoes CT.

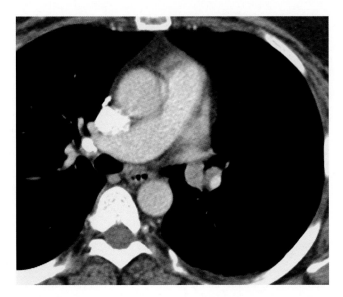

Figure 84.1

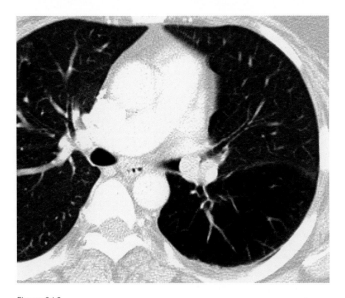

Figure 84.2

Case 84 Endobronchial Lesion (Carcinoid Tumor)

Figure 84.3

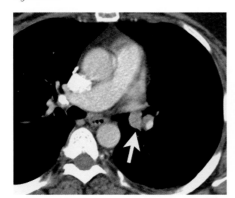

Figure 84.4

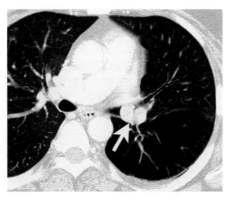

Findings

► CT demonstrates a soft tissue mass with moderate enhancement in the left mainstem bronchus (arrow in Fig. 84.3). The mass extends into and occludes the origin of the right lower lobe bronchus.

► Lung windows (Fig. 84.4) reveal hyperlucency of the left lobe due to air trapping.

Differential Diagnosis

► The differential diagnosis for an endobronchial lesion in an adult should be considered malignant until proven otherwise. It consists mainly of carcinoid tumor, squamous cell cancer, metastases, and rarely minor salivary gland tumors (mucoepidermoid and adenoid cystic tumors). Even more rarely, granulation tissue and hamartomas may present as endobronchial lesions.

Teaching Points

► Endobronchial carcinoids are neuroendocrine tumors that originate from the Kulchitsky cells in the bronchial and bronchiolar epithelium.

► Bronchial carcinoids represent 1% to 2% of all lung tumors.

► Carcinoid tumors are subdivided into typical and atypical, based on histology. Typical carcinoids show minimal mitoses; atypical carcinoids demonstrate necrosis or 2 to 10 mitoses per 10 high-power fields. 80% to 90% of carcinoid tumors are typical carcinoid tumors and the remaining 10% to 20% are atypical carcinoid tumors.

► Carcinoid tumors can secrete serotonin, adrenocorticotropic hormone (ACTH), somatostatin, and bradykinin; patients rarely present with syndromes related to ectopic hormone production of ACTH or Cushing syndrome. Carcinoid syndrome occurs only when there are liver metastases.

► CT shows a round, lobulated, well-circumscribed mass, closely associated with the bronchus. The tumor can be mostly outside the airway with only a small endoluminal portion, creating a "tip of the iceberg" sign.

► Carcinoids commonly obstruct the airway. Post-obstructive parenchymal changes vary from air trapping to atelectasis and lobar collapse with post-obstructive pneumonia. Mucous impaction in the distal bronchi may create mucoceles and tree-in-bud nodules.

► Carcinoid tumors commonly show eccentric calcification, a feature not easily identifiable by conventional radiography.

► Even though carcinoid tumors are highly vascular lesions, CT demonstrates variable degrees of enhancement.

Management

► All carcinoids are treated by surgical resection, because both typical and atypical carcinoids have a potential for metastasis.

Further Reading

Jeung MY, Gasser B, Gangi A, et al. Bronchial carcinoid tumors of the thorax: spectrum of radiologic findings. *Radiographics*. 2002 Mar-Apr; 22(2):351-365.

History

► 42-year-old woman with recurrent pneumonia and hemoptysis undergoes chest radiography followed by CT.

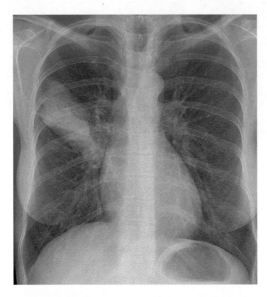

Figure 85.1

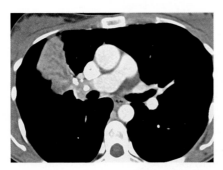

Figure 85.2a

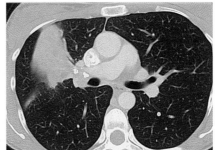

Figure 85.2b

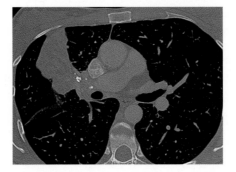

Figure 85.2c

Case 85 Broncholithiasis

Figure 85.3

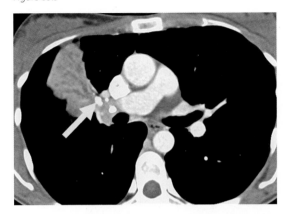

Findings

▶ Chest radiograph (Fig. 85.1) demonstrates partial collapse of the right upper lobe and calcifications in the right hilum.

▶ CT (Fig. 85.2 a–c) shows a densely calcified lesion, centered over the right upper lobe bronchus (arrow in Fig. 85.3), with distal mucus plugging of the segmental bronchi and associated atelectasis. A second calcified lymph node in the right hilum is noted.

Differential Diagnosis

▶ The differential diagnosis for partial lobar collapse from a very high-attenuating structure consists mainly of a foreign body or a broncholith. Rarely, carcinoid tumors may briskly enhance and simulate a broncholith. Because of the other calcifications, broncholithiasis would be favored.

Teaching Points

▶ A broncholith is a calcified or ossified object in the bronchus, which leads to obstruction of the bronchus.

▶ Most are formed by either erosion or extrusion of calcified peribronchial lymph nodes into the bronchial lumen. In situ calcification of aspirated foreign material is another way a broncholith can develop.

▶ Symptoms are nonproductive cough, hemoptysis, and less commonly post-obstructive pneumonia. Lithoptosis (coughing of stones), although rare, may happen.

▶ On CT, a broncholith appears as a calcified endobronchial lesion that has sharp edges or spurs, creating a typical irregular shape. Various manifestations of airway obstruction are seen, which include atelectasis, bronchiectasis, mucus plugging, pneumonia, and expiratory air trapping.

▶ Thin collimation, multiplanar reformations, and viewing with a bone window setting are helpful measures to assess the location, morphology, and density.

Management

▶ Broncholiths are removed when they cause repeated hemoptysis or infection. The preferred method is segmentectomy or lobectomy, since removal of the broncholith alone does not resolve the bronchial stenosis caused by the longstanding inflammation, leading to continued distal atelectasis and pneumonia.

▶ Bronchoscopic removal is difficult and commonly associated with catastrophic hemorrhage, because commonly a component of the lesion traverses the bronchial wall. In anticipation of severe hemorrhage, a rigid bronchoscope should be used.

Further Reading

Seo JB, Song KS, Lee JS, et al. Broncholithiasis: review of the causes with radiologic-pathologic correlation. *Radiographics*. 2002 Oct; 22 Spec No: S199-213.

History

▶ 51-year-old man with a nonproductive cough. He has also noted an unintentional 13-pound weight loss during the past few months.

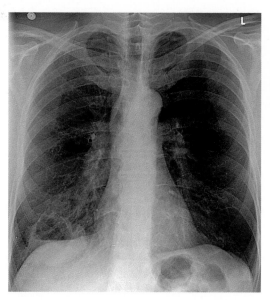

Figure 86.1

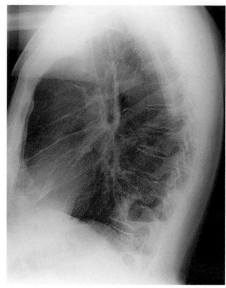

Figure 86.2

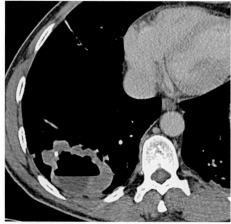

Figure 86.3

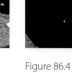

Figure 86.4

Case 86   Squamous Cell Carcinoma of the Lung

Figure 86.5

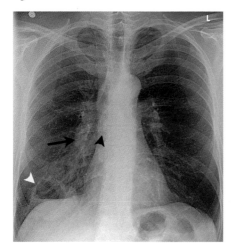

Figure 86.6

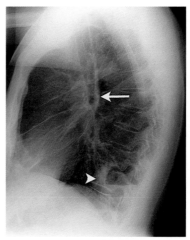

Findings

▶ Chest radiograph shows a cavity containing an air-fluid level in the right lower lobe (white arrowheads in Figs. 86.5 and 86.6). Right hilar lymphadenopathy (black arrow in Fig. 86.5) and subcarinal lymphadenopathy (black arrowhead in Fig. 86.5) are also seen. Thickening of the posterior wall of the bronchus intermedius (white arrow in **Fig.** 86.6) is suggestive of mediastinal lymphadenopathy.

▶ CT (Figs. 86.3 and 86.4) reveals irregular thick wall of this cavity and mediastinal and right hilar lymphadenopathy.

Differential Diagnosis

▶ Cavitary lung lesions can be secondary to infections (bacteria, fungi, parasites), neoplasm (primary or metastatic disease), trauma, vasculitis (c-ANCA-positive vasculitis), or congenital lung lesions (sequestrations). The presence of one dominant lesion with extensive lymphadenopathy would make lung cancer the main concern in this case.

Teaching Points

▶ *Cavity* is used for an oval or round lesion that contains air and has a wall thickness >4 mm. The term is employed for air developing within consolidation or a mass.

▶ Both lung cancer and lung abscess commonly have thick walls with irregular inner margins and lobulated or ill-defined outer margins. Air-fluid levels and hilar and mediastinal lymphadenopathy can be seen with both entities. The CT finding of a wall thickness >8 mm is suggestive of lung cancer.

▶ Up to 16% of lung cancers present as a cavity. Cavitation at presentation is associated with a worse prognosis, even at stage I disease. Central necrosis is due to rapid growth of the lesions, exceeding the blood supply.

▶ Most cavitating primary lung cancers are squamous cell carcinomas.

Management

▶ Management of a solitary cavitary mass depends on its etiology. Diagnosis may require biopsy to differentiate lung cancer from a cavitary indolent infection. If the pulmonary lesion is biopsied, care should be taken to sample the wall of the lesion, not the internal necrotic material.

Further Reading

Onn A, Choe DH, Herbst RS, et al. Tumor cavitation in stage I non-small cell lung cancer: epidermal growth factor receptor expression and prediction of poor outcome. *Radiology*. 2005 Oct;237(1):342-347.

History

▶ 50-year-old neutropenic woman with leukemia develops a fever.

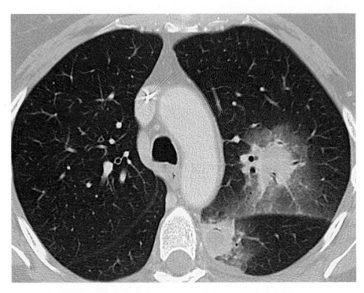

Figure 87.1

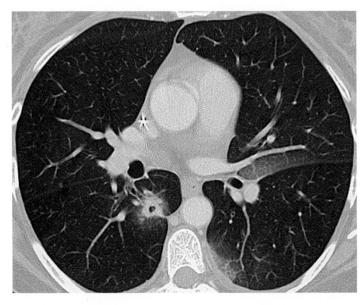

Figure 87.2

Case 87 Angioinvasive Aspergillus

Figure 87.3

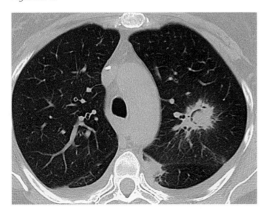

Findings

▶ CT (Figs. 87.1 and 87.2) shows multiple nodules bilaterally, some of which have internal cavitation. All of the nodules demonstrate adjacent ground-glass rims or halos.

Differential Diagnosis

▶ The main differential is based on the identification of multiple nodules with ground-glass halos, signifying adjacent hemorrhage or volume-averaging of lesion infiltration into
normal lung. Most cases of nodules with halos are from fungal infection (most notably angioinvasive aspergillus), hemorrhagic metastases (such as melanoma or angiosarcoma),
or vasculitis. The clinical history of neutropenia forced us to consider angioinvasive aspergillus first.

Teaching Points

▶ Angioinvasive aspergillosis (AIA) is the most common fungal infection in immunocompromised patients.
▶ Mucormycosis may also present with angioinvasion and subsequent ground-glass halos.
▶ AIA leads to ischemic necrosis and parenchymal infarction. The surrounding alveolar hemorrhage creates the halo.
▶ Since serologic tests of AIA, such as galactomannan, become positive late and sputum samples are not reliable, the CT halo sign may be the only reliable means of early diagnosis in a febrile, neutropenic patient.
▶ AIA occurs most frequently with bone marrow transplantation and hematological malignancies, and much less frequently in those with impaired cell-mediated immunity, such patients who have undergone lung, kidney, or heart transplantation.
▶ A characteristic CT finding is multiple nodules measuring 1 to 3 cm in diameter, with surrounding halos.
▶ The air crescent sign is a term that is often confused with mycetoma. It was originally described as a finding of healing angioinvasive aspergillus. The air crescent sign is usually seen 2 to 3 weeks after initiating therapy. It is caused by contraction of the central infarcted tissue, creating a crescentic space between it and the surrounding viable parenchyma (Fig. 87.3).

Management

▶ Antifungal therapy is usually initiated, with a 50% to 60% response rate to antifungal therapy. Response rate improves with earlier initiation of therapy.
▶ Biopsy is usually not performed as many of the neutropenic patients tend to be thrombocytopenic as well.

Further Reading

Franquet T, Müller NL, Giménez A, et al. Spectrum of pulmonary aspergillosis: histologic, clinical, and radiologic findings. *Radiographics*. 2001 Jul-Aug; 21(4):825-837.

History

▶ 72-year-old woman with productive cough receives this chest CT to evaluate nodules seen on recent chest radiograph.

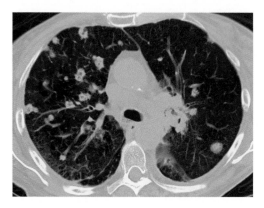

Figure 88.1

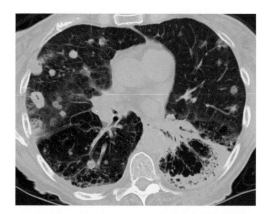

Figure 88.2

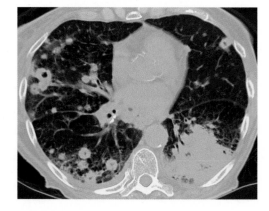

Figure 88.3

Case 88 Multifocal Bronchioloalveolar Carcinoma (Minimally Invasive Adenocarcinoma)

Findings

► CT shows multiple soft tissue nodules, many of which have central cavitation, as well as a large area of cavitary consolidation in the left lower lobe.

Differential Diagnosis

► Bronchioloalveolar carcinoma (BAC), metastatic disease (especially adenocarcinomas), and c-ANCA vasculitis can all present with these findings.

Teaching Points

► BAC accounts for 20% of primary lung cancers and may appear as a focal nodule, focal ground-glass opacity, persistent consolidation, or multifocal disease. While true cavitation can occur, pseudocavitation is more common, from the lepidic growth of the tumor, preserving the normal lung architecture and leaving distal bronchioles/alveolar sacs free of disease.

► The finding of soft tissue nodules with clean central cavitation is referred to as a "Cheerio" sign. BAC is in this differential diagnosis due to central pseudocavitation. Mucinous adenocarcinomas, frequently from the pancreas or gastrointestinal tract, c-ANCA vasculitis, and pulmonary Langerhans cell histiocytosis can also present with the Cheerio sign.

► As BAC frequently shows low metabolic activity, FDG-PET may be falsely negative. Consolidative forms mimic pneumonia and persist despite antibiotic treatment.

► Despite extensive radiographic disease, many patients have relatively few symptoms. While rare, bronchorrhea, persistent sputum production, can be seen, especially in mucinous types.

► Recent changes in lung cancer staging and classification have promoted the termination of *BAC* in favor of *minimally invasive adenocarcinoma and adenocarcinoma in-situ*, reflecting the ambiguity of the term *BAC* and frequent overlap with more aggressive tumors.

Management

► For nodular forms, CT-guided biopsy can be used to establish the diagnosis. If there is a mixture of ground-glass and soft tissue attenuation, preferential sampling of the soft tissue component may demonstrate frank adenocarcinoma.

► Consolidative forms can either be approached with transbronchial or CT-guided biopsy.

► While isolated nodular disease has a good prognosis, multifocal forms of disease have 5-year survival rates <50%, leading to the changes in terminology alluded to above.

Further Reading

Lee KS, Kim Y, Han J, et al. Bronchoalveolar carcinoma: clinical, histopathologic, and radiologic findings. *Radiographics.* 1997 Nov-Dec;17(6):1345-1357.

Patsios D, Roberts HC, Paul NS, et al. Pictorial review of the many faces of bronchoalveolar carcinoma. *Br J Radiol.* 2007 Dec;80(960): 1015-1023.

Part 12   Diffuse Lung Disease

Case 89

History

- 28-year-old woman with known cardiac disease presents with dyspnea.

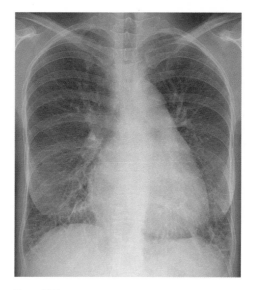

Figure 89.1

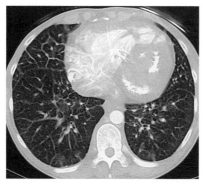

Figure 89.2

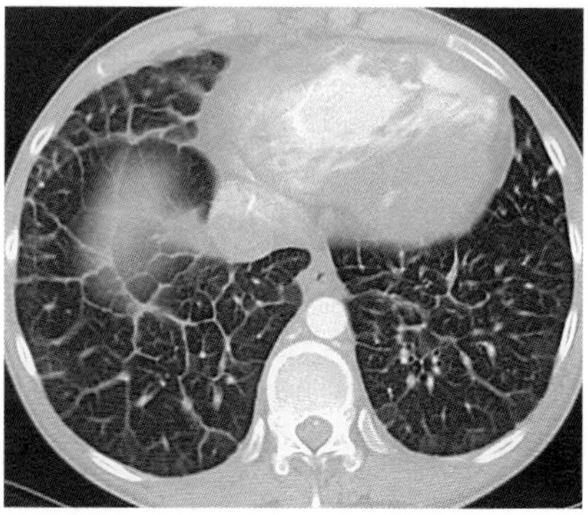

Figure 89.3

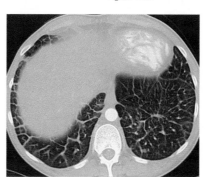

Figure 89.4

Case 89 Cardiogenic Pulmonary Edema

Figure 89.5

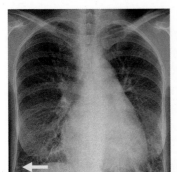

Figure 89.6

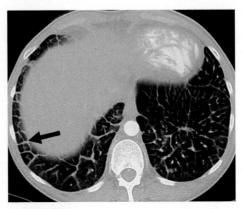

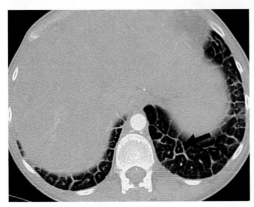

Figure 89.7

Findings

► Chest radiograph shows bilateral septal lines (Kerley B lines) (arrow in Fig. 89.5).
► CT confirmed smooth interlobular septal line thickening (arrow in Fig. 89.6). The smooth septal lines outline the secondary pulmonary lobules (arrow in Fig. 89.7).

Differential Diagnosis

► The differential diagnosis for smooth septal line thickening is based on acuity. Acutely, smooth septal lines are usually seen in hydrostatic or cardiogenic edema. They can also be seen in hemorrhage (which usually has accompanying ground glass) or viral pneumonias (which usually have ground-glass nodules). More chronic smooth septal line thickening can be seen with lymphangitic carcinomatosis and, very rarely, amyloid or lymphoma. Given the history of cardiac disease, cardiogenic edema should be favored.

Teaching Points

► Hydrostatic pulmonary edema refers to the presence of interstitial fluid within the lungs, usually from left heart failure (cardiogenic pulmonary edema). Other causes include isolated pulmonary venous obstruction, fluid overload, and hypoalbuminemia.
► Pleural effusions and cardiomegaly may be seen in cardiogenic edema.
► Radiographic findings of cardiogenic edema include interlobular septal line thickening, peribronchial cuffing, ground-glass opacities, and frank consolidation.

- Cardiogenic pulmonary edema does not follow a programmed course from interstitial edema to consolidation. Patients can present acutely with either interstitial or airspace disease.
- Peripheral 1 to 2-cm interlobular septal lines are sometimes referred to as Kerley B lines. Kerley A lines are central interlobular septal lines that are longer.
- Cardiogenic edema is usually bilateral. Unilateral edema should prompt inspection of central structures to look for a mass that may be compressing the pulmonary vein. Most of the time, unilateral pulmonary edema develops because of patient positioning.
- Cardiogenic edema should clear rapidly as the patient improves clinically. When it does not change, alternative diagnoses should be considered, such as lymphangitic carcinomatosis or, in the setting of ground glass, diffuse alveolar damage.

Management

- Cardiogenic edema is usually treated with supportive therapy and diuretics. Once the patient is through the acute situation, attempts are made to maximize cardiac function.

Further Reading

Webb WR. Thin-section CT of the secondary pulmonary lobule: anatomy and the image: the 2004 Fleischner lecture. *Radiology*. 2006 May;239(2):322-338.

History

▶ 65-year-old man presents with sudden onset of shortness of breath.

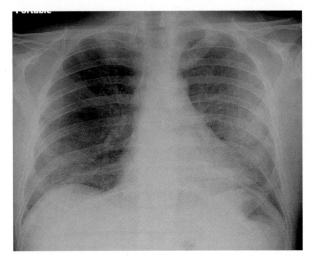

Figure 90.1

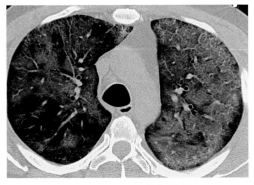

Figure 90.2

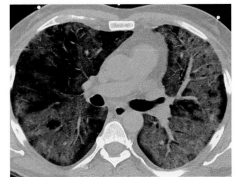

Figure 90.3

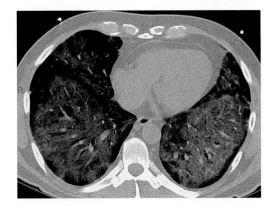

Figure 90.4

Case 90 Noncardiogenic Edema Pattern (Acute Interstitial Pneumonia)

Figure 90.5

Figure 90.6

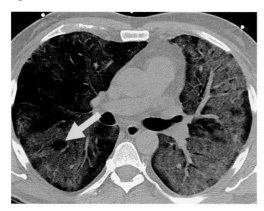
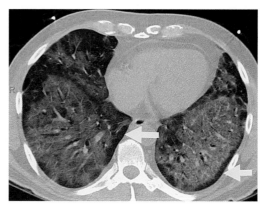

Findings

▶ Chest radiograph (Fig. 90.1) shows bilateral airspace disease that is greater on the left. No pleural effusion or cardiac enlargement is seen.

▶ CT shows bilateral ground-glass opacities with secondary lobular sparing (arrow in Fig. 90.5) and relative peripheral sparing (arrows in Fig. 90.6). Note the visualization of few dilated bronchi in Figure 90.6. Few interlobular septal lines are seen in isolation.

Differential Diagnosis

▶ The differential diagnosis for this diffuse pattern is headed by pulmonary edema. The lack of pleural effusions, normal cardiac size, peripheral sparing, and absence of interlobular septal lines makes hydrostatic edema (cardiogenic edema) less likely. The findings are more suggestive of a permeative (noncardiogenic) pattern. Without any known cause, one would wonder about idiopathic-onset adult respiratory distress syndrome (ARDS), also known as acute interstitial pneumonia (AIP).

Teaching Points

▶ Noncardiogenic edema or edema from increased permeability can be associated with diffuse alveolar damage and the clinical diagnosis of ARDS.

▶ Noncardiogenic edema with diffuse alveolar damage is less likely to present with Kerley B lines and more likely to present with air bronchograms. Other CT findings of ARDS include increased density of the lungs in dependent regions from increased atelectasis and secondary lobular sparing (which should not be confused for air-trapping).

▶ Edema from increased vascular permeability may be seen in a variety of conditions, including inhalation injuries, trauma, high altitude, shock, drugs, and neurologic disease. Often these conditions will have an element of diffuse alveolar damage.

▶ Noncardiogenic edema without alveolar damage may be seen as the result of a transfusion reaction or a drug reaction.

▶ Occasionally, edema will be from a mixed hydrostatic and increased permeability pattern. This mixed pattern may be seen in neurogenic edema, high-altitude edema, re-expansion edema, post-lobectomy/pneumonectomy edema, illicit drug-induced edema (crack, cocaine), and post-transplant edema.

Management

▶ In AIP and ARDS, treatment is supportive.

Further Reading

Lynch DA, Travis WD, Müller NL, et al. Idiopathic interstitial pneumonias: CT features. *Radiology*. 2005 Jul;236(1):10-21.

History

▶ 55-year-old woman presents with 1 month of dyspnea. She receives a radiograph (Fig. 91.1) followed by CT (Figs. 91.3 and 91.4).

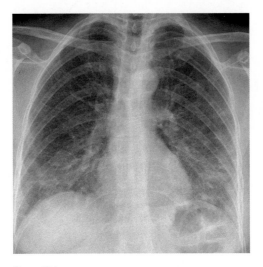

Figure 91.1

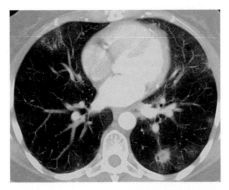

Figure 91.2

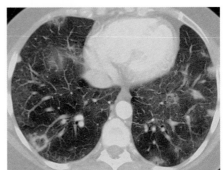

Figure 91.3

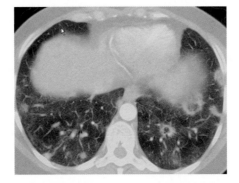
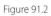

Figure 91.4

Case 91 Organizing Pneumonia

Figure 91.5

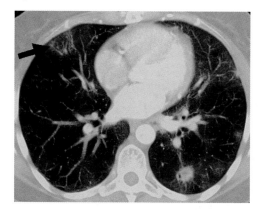

Figure 91.6

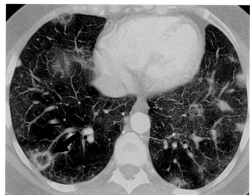

Findings

► Chest radiograph (Fig. 91.1) shows bilateral airspace disease greater on the left and in the bases. No pleural effusion or cardiac enlargement is seen.

► CT shows bilateral ground-glass opacities and nodules. Many of the nodules touch the pleural surfaces and some are crescentic (arrow in Fig. 91.5). This has been referred to as an *atoll sign* because its appearance is similar to that of a coral atoll. Other nodular areas have an outer more solid-appearing ring with internal ground glass (arrow in Fig. 91.6), or *reverse halo*. Current recommendations prefer the use of *reverse halo*.

Differential Diagnosis

► Differential diagnosis for the reverse halo sign includes vasculitis (such as Churg-Strauss or Wegener's granulomatosis), infection (fungal, most notably paracoccidioidomycosis), angioinvasive lymphoma, and organizing pneumonia (OP).

Teaching Points

► OP is a nonspecific pattern of organization of fibroblasts and inflammatory cells in response to acute lung injury.

► Recently, *OP* has gained favor over other names such as bronchiolitis obliterans organizing pneumonia (BOOP) to avoid any confusion with bronchiolitis obliterans—a completely different entity.

► *Cryptogenic OP* (COP) is usually reserved for cases of OP that are idiopathic.

► OP may be secondary to infection, drug and toxin injury, collagen vascular disease, hypersensitivity pneumonitis, chronic eosinophilic pneumonia, vasculitis, or neoplasm.

► The most common patterns of OP on CT are ground-glass opacity and consolidation. Often the airspace changes are seen in a peribronchovascular or subpleural location. Pleural effusions are characteristically absent.

► The reverse halo sign is seen in <20% of patients with OP.

► Patients tend to present with low-grade fevers, mild dyspnea, and malaise.

► When chronic eosinophilic pneumonia (CEP) is biopsied, large areas of OP are often encountered. This feature may help to explain the overlap in CT features between OP and CEP.

Management

► Most cases of COP are responsive to corticosteroids, making OP one of the few reversible manifestations of lung injury.

Further Reading

Kim SJ, Lee KS, Ryu YH, et al. Reversed halo sign on high-resolution CT of cryptogenic organizing pneumonia: diagnostic implications. *AJR Am J Roentgenol.* 2003 May;180:1251-1254.

History

▶ 80-year-old woman with persistent cough is treated for pneumonia. When the follow-up radiograph is unchanged, she undergoes a chest CT.

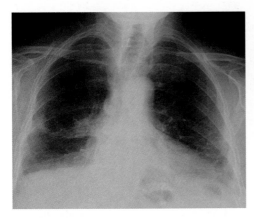

Figure 92.1

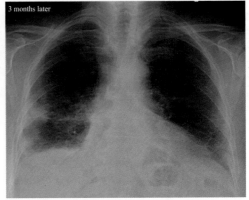

Figure 92.2

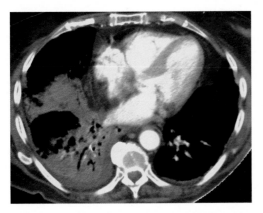

Figure 92.3

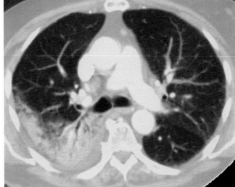

Figure 92.4

Case 92   Bronchioloalveolar Cell Carcinoma (BAC) (Minimally Invasive Adenocarcinoma)

Figure 92.5

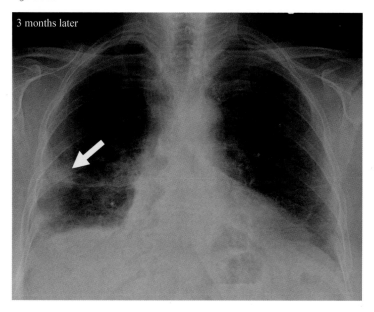

Findings

► Persistent consolidation (white arrow in Fig. 92.5) is seen in the periphery of the right lung base.
► CT demonstrates right middle lobe and right lower lobe consolidation with air bronchograms and unaffected pulmonary vessels in the consolidation (*CT angiogram sign*).

Differential Diagnosis

► For persistent consolidation, the differential diagnosis would include bronchioloalveolar cell carcinoma (BAC), lymphoma, organizing pneumonia, eosinophilic pneumonia, atypical infection (such as a fungal pneumonia), or a congenital lesion (such as sequestration)

Teaching Points

► Persistent consolidation, despite interval treatment, on chest radiographs should prompt expansion of the differential diagnosis beyond routine pneumonia. First, a post-obstructive cause should be considered due to a central bronchogenic malignancy, endobronchial lesion such as carcinoid tumor, hilar adenopathy, or broncholithiasis. CT is often the next step in evaluation.
► If no obstructing central mass is seen, atypical infections not covered by routine antibiotics, especially fungal infections, should be considered.
► BAC, most commonly the mucinous form, presents as consolidation in approximately 30% of cases. An adenocarcinoma with intra-alveolar spread, BAC does not disturb the underlying architecture of the lung; rather, it fills the alveolar spaces with mucin and debris. Lymphoma, especially the mucosa-associated lymphatic tissue (MALT) form, can rarely present as focal consolidation.
► Organizing pneumonia is often seen as peripheral consolidation as a nonspecific response to lung injury.

► Eosinophilic pneumonia (especially the chronic form) can simulate organizing pneumonia but tends to have an upper lung predilection.
► CT can also be used to exclude a feeding vessel from the aorta to the consolidation to exclude pulmonary sequestration.

Management

► Bronchoscopy with lavage and/or transbronchial biopsy is usually the first route for diagnosis.
► BAC will be treated based on stage and whether any nonmucinous or high-grade lesions are present.

Further Reading

Lee KS, Kim Y, Han J, et al. Bronchoalveolar carcinoma: clinical, histopathologic, and radiologic findings. *Radiographics*. 1997 Nov-Dec;17(6):1345-1357.
Patsios D, Roberts HC, Paul NS, et al. Pictorial review of the many faces of bronchoalveolar cell carcinoma. *Br J Radiol*. 2007 Dec;80(960):1015-1023.

History

▶ 55-year-old man with progressive dyspnea on exertion undergoes CT for evaluation.

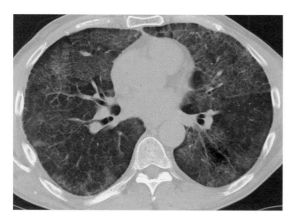

Figure 93.1

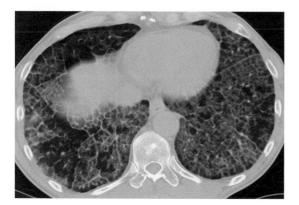

Figure 93.2

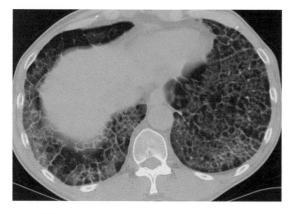

Figure 93.3

Case 93   Pulmonary Alveolar Proteinosis (with Crazy Paving)

Findings

▸ CT shows lower lung-predominant ground-glass attenuation and smooth septal line thickening. This combination is known as *crazy paving*. Note the absence of cardiac enlargement or pleural effusions.

Differential Diagnosis

▸ The differential diagnosis for crazy paving without pleural effusions includes noncardiogenic pulmonary edema, pneumocystis infection, pulmonary alveolar proteinosis (PAP), or drug or hypersensitivity reaction.

Teaching Points

▸ Frequently presenting with an indolent course and nonspecific complaints including dyspnea, PAP results from accumulation of periodic acid-Schiff-positive lipoproteinaceous surfactant material in the alveolar spaces.

▸ While PAP can be secondary in the setting of hematologic malignancies and certain particulate exposures, the majority of cases are considered primary and recent studies suggest an autoimmune component involving GM-CSF.

▸ While the crazy paving pattern is commonly associated with PAP, it is nonspecific and can be seen in cardiogenic pulmonary edema, pulmonary hemorrhage syndromes, atypical infections, lipoid pneumonia, diffuse alveolar damage, mucinous bronchoalveolar carcinoma, and drug or hypersensitivity reactions. Lack of pleural effusions and absence of cardiomegaly should lead the reader to consider noncardiogenic causes of this pattern.

▸ In cases of PAP, the radiographic findings are often more dramatic than the clinical symptoms.

▸ Lipoid pneumonia, which results from the aspiration of exogenous lipoproteinaceous material, can simulate the crazy paving of PAP, but often lipoid pneumonia will have consolidation containing macroscopic fat.

Management

▸ Diagnosis is usually made by bronchoalveolar lavage. Rarely transbronchial biopsy or open lung biopsy will be performed. The finding of periodic acid-Schiff-positive lipoproteinaceous material allows for establishment of the diagnosis.

▸ PAP is usually self-limiting. Some patients will require whole lung lavage to alleviate symptoms until the disease begins to mitigate.

Further Reading

Holbert JM, Costello P, Li W, et al. CT features of pulmonary alveolar proteinosis. *AJR Am J Roentgenol.* 2001; 176:1287-1294.

Huizar I, Kavuru MS. Alveolar proteinosis syndrome: pathogenesis, diagnosis, and management. *Curr Opin Pulm Med.* 2009 Sep;15(5):491-498.

Rossi SE, Erasmus JJ, Volpacchio M, et al. "Crazy-paving" pattern at thin-section CT of the lungs: radiologic-pathologic overview. *Radiographics.* 2003 Nov-Dec; 23(6):1509-1519.

History

▶ 41-year-old man presents with basilar consolidation.

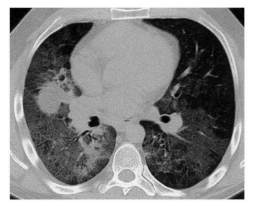

Figure 94.1

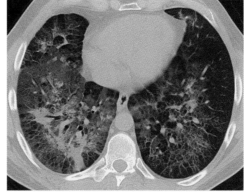

Figure 94.2

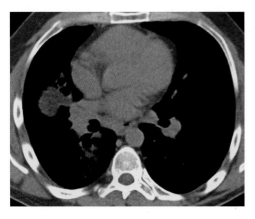

Figure 94.3

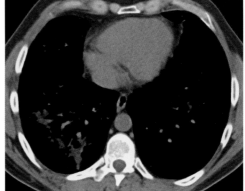

Figure 94.4

Case 94   Lipoid Pneumonia

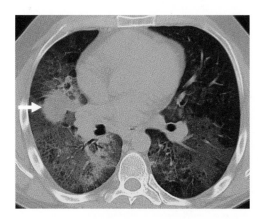

Figure 94.5

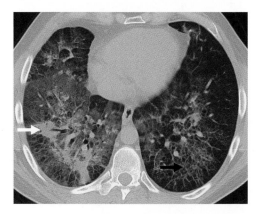

Figure 94.6

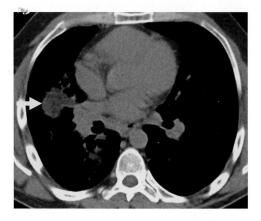

Figure 94.7

Findings

▶ Multiple areas of consolidation (white arrows in Figs. 94.5–94.7) are seen in the right middle and lower lobes, which have fat density on soft tissue windows. In addition, there is basilar ground-glass opacification and septal line thickening (*crazy paving*) (black arrow in Fig. 94.6).

Differential Diagnosis

▶ The key to this case is the identification of fat attenuation in the lung. This should prompt consideration of lipoid pneumonia or hamartoma. Only the former would present with crazy paving and consolidation.

Teaching Points

▶ While uncommon, exogenous lipoid pneumonia is most often encountered in older patients with oropharyngeal dysmotility in the setting of mineral oil laxative use or oils used to moisten lips or nasal airways.

▶ As a result of ensuing chemical pneumonitis, especially in the exposure to animal fats, acute lipoid pneumonia usually presents symptomatically with dyspnea and finding of airspace consolidation, ground glass, septal line thickening, and pleural effusions on CT imaging. Acute episodes most commonly resolve, possibly with residual scarring.

▶ Chronic lipoid pneumonia is usually detected incidentally on radiographs or imaging and has a similar appearance on CT as acute lipoid pneumonia, with the general exception of lack of pleural effusions. As fibrosis develops around the areas of lipoid material, the consolidation can mimic a primary pulmonary malignancy or atypical infection and can be FDG-avid on PET exams. Chronic lipoid pneumonia typically persists unchanged over time.

▶ Areas of fat throughout the consolidation are diagnostic of exogenous lipoid pneumonia. However, in the setting of acute inflammation, the fat attenuation can be masked secondary to averaging with proteinaceous or alveolar debris.

▶ Occasionally, lipoid pneumonia can present with pulmonary nodules. Nodular lipoid pneumonia can be distinguished from another fat-containing lesion, the pulmonary hamartoma, by its borders. Usually, hamartomas are smooth bordered, while lipoid pneumonia tends to be more spiculated.

Management

▶ Cessation of exposure to the offending lipoid agent is often all that is required. In the acute setting, care is supportive.

Further Reading

Betancourt SL, Martinez-Jimenez S, Rossi SE, et al. Lipoid pneumonia: spectrum of clinical and radiologic manifestations. *AJR Am J Roetgenol.* 2010 Jan;194(1):103-109.

History

▶ 83-year-old African American woman with chronic arrhythmia receives this chest CT.

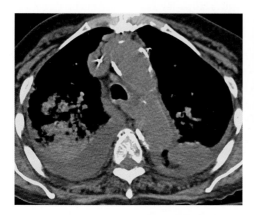

Figure 95.1

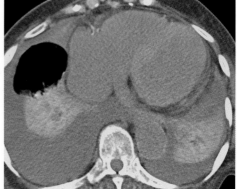

Figure 95.2

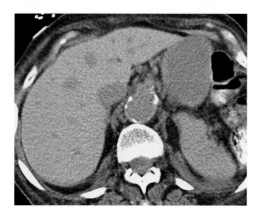

Figure 95.3

Case 95   Amiodarone Deposition

Findings

▶ Noncontrast CT shows high-density airspace opacities in the upper lungs (Fig. 95.1) and dense bibasilar atelectasis with small bilateral pleural effusions (Fig. 95.2). The liver parenchyma is also dense (Fig. 95.3).

Differential Diagnosis

▶ Amiodarone deposition, embolism of oil-based iodinated material (from lymphangiography or chemoembolization), amyloidosis, metastatic pulmonary calcification, and talcosis can present with high-attenuating lung parenchyma. Metastatic calcification may present with high-attenuation centrilobular nodules favoring the upper lungs.

Teaching Points

▶ Amiodarone hydrochloride is used for treatment of arrhythmias and contains iodine.

▶ Amiodarone deposition in the lung can result in high-attenuation consolidation because of the iodine.

▶ Amiodarone toxicity implies fibrotic and inflammatory change in the lung.Pulmonary toxicity may occur in up to 6% of patients receiving amiodarone. Most patients who develop toxicity have received doses at least 400 mg/d.

▶ Patients present with a gradual onset of shortness of breath, which begins several months after starting therapy. They rarely present with fever and acute dyspnea.

▶ CT manifestations of pulmonary involvement are varied and, consist of diffuse interstitial thickening; dense subpleural, wedge-shaped consolidations (organizing pneumonia); hyperdense atelectasis, and focal, round consolidations of high density. The density of affected lung ranges between 80 and 175 HU and is due to incorporation of the iodine into the type II pneumocytes.

▶ Homogenously high attenuation of liver parenchyma is common and is seen more often than high attenuation of the lung.

Management

▶ Management is based on whether toxicity is suspected over simple deposition. This decision is based on symptoms and evidence of organ compromise.

▶ When toxicity is suspected, therapy consists of cessation, with good prognosis. The half-life of amiodarone hydrochloride is approximately 30 days, so at least 1 month has to transpire to achieve clinical and radiographic resolution.

Further Reading

Ellis SJ, Cleverley JR, Müller NL. Drug-induced lung disease: high-resolution CT findings. *AJR Am J Roentgenol.* 2000;175:1019-1024.

Marchiori E, Souza AS, Franquet T, et al. Diffuse high-attenuation pulmonary abnormalities: a pattern-oriented diagnostic approach on high-resolution CT. *AJR Am J Roentgenol.* 2005;184:273-282.

Muller NL, Fraser RS, Colman NC, Paré PD (Eds.). Chapter 17: Drugs, Poisons, Irradiation. In *Radiologic Diagnosis of Diseases of the Chest*, 1st ed. Philadelphia: W.B. Saunders, 2001:571.

History

▶ 59-year-old man presents with chronic cough.

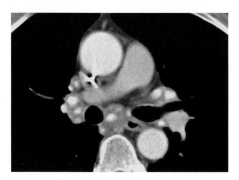

Figure 96.1

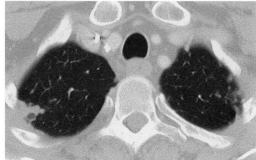

Figure 96.2

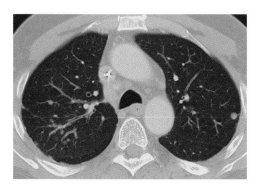

Figure 96.3

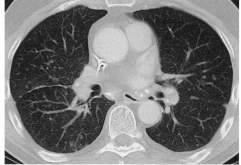

Figure 96.4

Case 96 Sarcoidosis with Perilymphatic Nodules

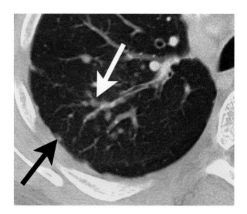

Figure 96.5

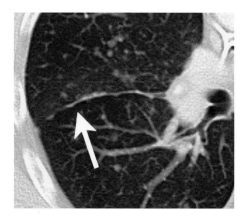

Figure 96.6

Findings

▶ CT demonstrates multiple calcified and enlarged mediastinal and right hilar lymph nodes (Fig. 96.1).

▶ Multiple subcentimeter nodules in the lungs, are located adjacent to the bronchovascular bundles (white arrow in Fig. 96.5), pleura (black arrow in Fig. 96.5), and fissures (white arrow in Fig. 96.6).

▶ The peripheral nodules coalesce in the apices (Fig. 96.2).

Differential Diagnosis

▶ The main differential diagnosis of perilymphatic nodules, especially with a predilection for the upper and middle lung, consists of sarcoidosis, silicosis, and coal-worker pneumoconiosis. The latter two are suspected when a relevant occupational history is discovered. Lymphangitic carcinomatosis may also present with perilymphatic nodules but tends to have more septal line thickening.

Teaching Points

▶ Perilymphatic distribution refers to nodules that involve the axial lymphatics, resulting in centrilobular and peribronchovascular findings, and the peripheral lymphatics, leading to abnormalities of the interlobular septa, fissures, and visceral pleura.

- Sarcoidosis is a granulomatous disease of unknown cause.
- Up to 60% of those affected with sarcoidosis are asymptomatic despite diffuse disease. Cough and dyspnea are the most common complaints.
- Histologic examination reveals non-necrotizing (or noncaseating) granulomas, located mostly along the lymphatics of the bronchovascular sheath, and to a lesser extent the subpleural and septal lymphatics.
- Nodules are seen on CT and HRCT of >80% of cases. These nodules are mostly 1 to 2 mm (micronodules) in diameter and ill defined. They represent aggregates of granulomas. Larger, more well-defined nodules, 3 mm to 1 cm in size, are also common.
- The findings are typically bilateral but may be asymmetric. Upper lung distribution is typical with both sarcoidosis and silicosis.
- Mediastinal and hilar lymphadenopathy, commonly calcified, is typically present. The calcification can be central, diffuse, or peripheral (eggshell).

Management

- Corticosteroids are the cornerstone of treating symptomatic or progressive sarcoidosis.
- Lung transplantation is considered for end-stage fibrotic disease.

Further Reading

Lynch JP 3rd, Ma YL, Koss MN, et al. Pulmonary sarcoidosis. *Semin Respir Crit Care Med.* 2007 Feb; 28(1):53-74.

Raoof S, Amchentsev A, Vlahos I, et al. Pictorial essay: multinodular disease—a high-resolution CT scan diagnostic algorithm. *Chest.* 2006; 129:805-815.

History

▶ 47-year-old woman who smokes a half-pack of cigarettes per day presents with a persistent dry cough.

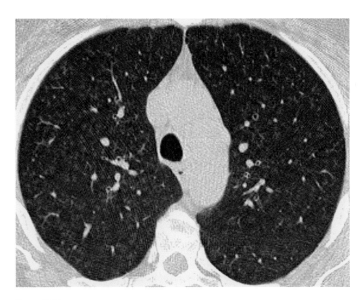

Figure 97.1

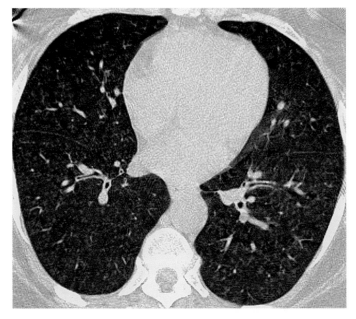

Figure 97.2

Case 97   Respiratory Bronchiolitis Interstitial Lung Disease (RB-ILD)

Figure 97.3

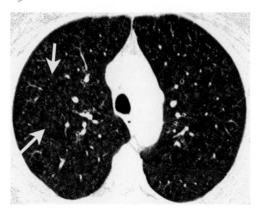

Findings

► CT images show diffuse tiny ground-glass centrilobular nodules without branching structures. In other words, this finding is not a tree-in-bud pattern. Viewing with narrower window settings makes these nodules more conspicuous (arrows in Fig. 97.3).

Differential Diagnosis

► Practically, the main differential diagnosis for centrilobular nodules on CT is respiratory bronchiolitis (RB), RB-ILD, or subacute hypersensitivity pneumonitis. The history of smoking would make the latter highly unlikely.

Teaching Points

► RB and RB-ILD are chronic diseases of heavy smokers in which pigmented macrophages accumulate in the respiratory bronchioles and mild peribronchial interstitial thickening develops.
► The process is called RB-ILD when the patient is symptomatic with cough or dyspnea.
► Most patients with RB-ILD have smoked for 30 years. Patients present between 30 and 50 years of age.
► 50% of patients with RB-ILD have bibasilar end-respiratory crackles. Pulmonary function tests (PFTs) can be normal or show a mixed restrictive-obstructive pattern.
► CT findings are typically subtle and characterized by multiple faint nodules of ground-glass opacity with ill-defined margins, measuring 3 to 5 mm in diameter. They are located in the center of the secondary pulmonary lobule (centrilobular or bronchocentric).
► RB-ILD can be diffuse or favor the upper lobes.
► Rarely, in end-stage renal disease, metastatic pulmonary calcification may present with ground-glass centrilobular nodules.

Management

► When centrilobular nodules are encountered on CT, the smoking history is solicited. If there is no history of smoking, hypersensitivity is favored. If the patient is a smoker, RB or RB-ILD is favored. RB and RB-ILD should improve with smoking cessation.
► Confirmatory diagnosis, which is almost never required, can be made with open or thoracoscopic biopsy.

Further Reading

Attili AK, Kazerooni EA, Gross BH, et al. Smoking-related interstitial lung disease: radiologic-clinical-pathologic correlation. *Radiographics.* 2008 Sep-Oct;28(5):1383-1396.
Park JS, Brown KK, Tuder RM, et al. Respiratory bronchiolitis-associated interstitial lung disease: radiologic features with clinical and pathologic correlation. *J Comput Assist Tomogr.* 2002 Jan-Feb;26(1):13-20.

History

▶ 89-year-old woman with respiratory failure receives this chest CT.

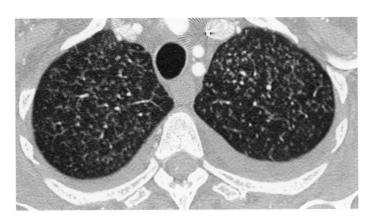

Figure 98.1

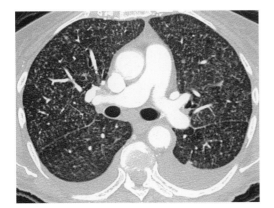

Figure 98.2

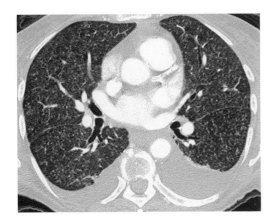

Figure 98.3

Case 98 Miliary Tuberculosis

Figure 98.4

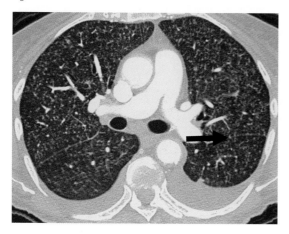

Findings

▸ Innumerable, diffuse micronodules are seen throughout the upper and lower lobes of both lungs. These nodules are best described as "random" as they affect the centrilobular structures and the pleural/fissural surfaces (arrow in Fig. 98.4). Small bilateral pleural effusions are also seen.

Differential Diagnosis

▸ Miliary infection (including fungal diseases, such as histoplasmosis, and mycobacterial disease, such as tuberculosis) and hematogenous metastases lead the differential diagnosis. Rarely, sarcoidosis can take on a miliary pattern.

Teaching Points

▸ Unlike perilymphatic nodules that also touch the pleural surfaces, miliary nodules are not clustered in regions of the lung; rather, they are uniformly distributed throughout the lungs. Reflecting hematogenous spread, miliary nodules may have a slight lower lung predominance due to the greater perfusion to the lower lobes.

▸ Miliary refers to the resemblance of these tiny nodules (1–3 mm in size) to millet seeds.

▸ Miliary nodules are present in slightly less than 10% of primary tuberculosis cases and are also seen in cases of reactivation tuberculosis.

▸ Disseminated fungal disease, such as histoplasmosis, can have a similar appearance.

▸ Certain malignancies, such as thyroid, renal, and melanoma, can produce innumerable micronodular metastases.

▸ Patients who are immunocompromised from diabetes, severe illness, debilitation, or HIV/AIDS are at risk for reactivation miliary tuberculosis.

Management

▸ Referring clinicians should be directly contacted whenever tuberculosis is in the differential diagnosis. Tree-in-bud opacities reflect endobronchial spread and these patients are at high risk of airborne transmission. Isolated miliary disease as a result of its hematogenous spread is not at risk of airborne spread.

▸ When miliary nodules are detected, blood cultures for tuberculosis should be performed. PPD may be placed. Sputum induction for acid-fast bacillus is usually not as helpful as it is with tree-in-bud nodules. Rarely, transbronchial biopsy is needed for diagnosis.

Further Reading

Jeong YJ, Lee KS. Pulmonary tuberculosis: up-to-date imaging and management. *AJR Am J Roentgenol.* 2008;191:834-844.
Raoof S, Amchentsev A, Vlahos I, et al. Pictorial essay: multinodular disease: a high-resolution CT scan diagnostic algorithm. *Chest.* 2006 Mar;129(3):805-815.

History

▶ 70-year-old woman with a nonproductive cough is referred for chest CT.

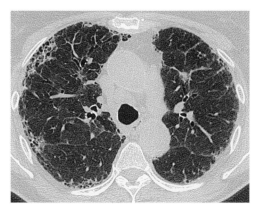

Figure 99.1

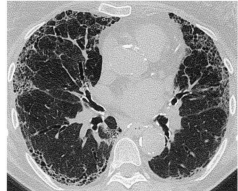

Figure 99.2

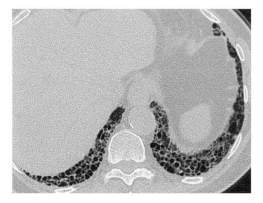

Figure 99.3

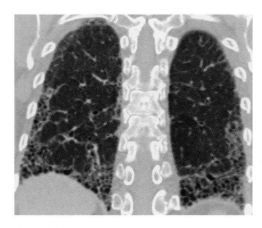

Figure 99.4

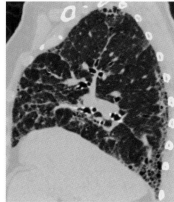

Figure 99.5

Case 99   Usual Interstitial Pneumonia (UIP) Pattern/Idiopathic Pulmonary Fibrosis (IPF)

Figure 99.6

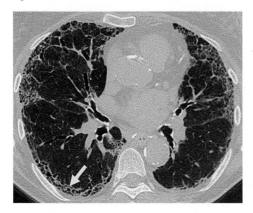

Findings

► CT images (Figs. 99.1–99.3) show interlobular septal thickening, architectural distortion, and traction bronchiectasis. The dominant pattern is honeycombing in the periphery and bases of the lungs (arrow in Fig. 99.6). Note the multiple rows of cysts, which allow for distinction from paraseptal emphysema, which usually consists of only one row of cysts.
► CT reconstructions (Figs. 99.4 and 99.5) clearly delineate the basilar predominance of disease.

Differential Diagnosis

► Based on the honeycombing, the differential diagnosis would be led by a usual interstitial pneumonitis (UIP) pattern of fibrosis. Other potential etiologies for the honeycombing would include asbestosis, rheumatoid arthritis, or chronic hypersensitivity. Given any findings to suggest these other entities, such as pleural plaques, shoulder arthritis, or air-trapping, idiopathic UIP would be favored.

Teaching Points

► UIP is the disease seen with idiopathic pulmonary fibrosis (IPF); most cases of UIP are idiopathic.
► Pathologic diagnosis is made by identifying fibroblastic foci with spatial and temporal heterogeneity of fibrosis.
► The incidence of IPF is slightly greater in male patients who are over 50 and smoke.
► UIP/IPF has an insidious onset and usually presents with 6 months of worsening dyspnea with dry basilar crackles.
► The mean survival rate from time of diagnosis is typically between 2 and 5 years.
► On HRCT, honeycombing is the strongest indicator of UIP pattern of fibrosis.
► The fibrotic changes are worst in the subpleural and lower lungs.
► IPF is associated with an increased incidence of lung cancer (10–15% of patients with IPF will develop lung cancer).
► Increasingly, radiologists are asked to describe the HRCT findings as a "pattern," highlighting the importance of clinical information in clinching the final diagnosis.

Management

► When the findings are typical, HRCT is a reliable means of diagnosis, prediction of response to therapy, and survival, thereby obviating the need for biopsy.
► Attempts to slow the rate of progression medically have not been successful.
► Lung transplantation is the treatment of choice for patients with progressive disease.

Further Reading

Lynch DA, Travis WD, Muller NL, et al. Idiopathic interstitial pneumonias: CT features. *Radiology*. 2005; 236:10-12.

History

▶ 49-year-old man presents with hemoptysis.

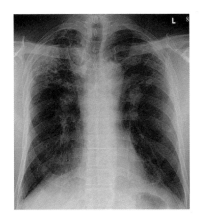

Figure 100.1

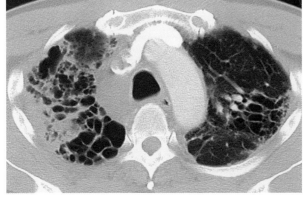

Figure 100.2

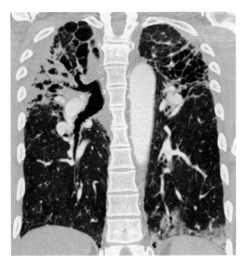

Figure 100.3

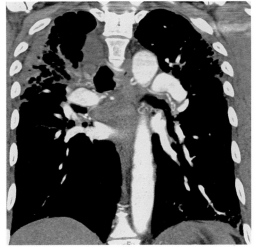

Figure 100.4

Case 100 Upper Lung Honeycombing (End-Stage Sarcoidosis)

Figure 100.5

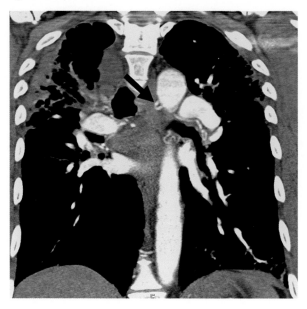

Findings

▶ Frontal chest radiograph shows reticulonodular opacities in the upper lungs with elevation of the hila and tenting of the diaphragm from upper lung volume loss.

▶ CT images (Figs. 100.2 and 100.3) demonstrate the cystic changes of honeycombing, bronchiectasis, and fibrotic mass-like densities.

▶ The enlarged lymph nodes and bronchial arteries (arrow in Fig. 100.5) are best displayed with soft-tissue settings.

Differential Diagnosis

▶ Upper lung pulmonary fibrosis with honeycombing and volume loss can be seen with end-stage sarcoidosis, silicosis, and scarring from prior infection (usually tuberculosis or histoplasmosis). End-stage hypersensitivity pneumonitis can sometimes have a similar distribution.

Teaching Points

▶ Sarcoidosis is overall the second most common cause of pulmonary fibrosis, after usual interstitial pneumonia. It develops about 10 years after initial diagnosis.

▶ Sarcoidosis involves the pulmonary parenchyma and mediastinal lymph nodes in 90% of cases. Most parenchymal findings resolve spontaneously or in response to corticosteroid treatment.

▶ 20% to 25% of pulmonary sarcoidosis cases progress to fibrosis, considered stage IV of disease. This is associated with increased morbidity and mortality.

▶ Imaging findings include reticular opacities of the upper lungs, associated with honeycombing and volume loss. The process is worse around the bronchovascular bundles, causing distortion and displacement of the fissures, bronchi, and vessels. Traction bronchiectasis and perilymphatic micronodules are common.

- Stage IV sarcoidosis shares features with silicosis in that it can have upper lung fibrotic masses >3 cm in diameter and eggshell calcification of the mediastinal and hilar lymph nodes. Paracicatricial emphysema adjacent to the massive fibrosis can be a site of saprophytic aspergillus infection with mycetoma formation.
- Bronchial arteries may become dilated in the setting of severe fibrosis. These collateral arteries are friable and commonly cause hemoptysis. Bronchial artery hypertrophy is less common in usual interstitial pneumonia.

Management

- There is no treatment of stage IV sarcoidosis. Pulmonary transplantation may be considered. Recurrence of sarcoidosis in the transplanted lung can occur.

Further Reading

Abehsera M, Valeyre D, Grenier P, et al. Sarcoidosis with pulmonary fibrosis: CT patterns and correlation with pulmonary function. *AJR Am J Roentgenol.* 2000 Jun;174(6):1751-1757.

Primack SL, Hartman TE, Hansell DM, et al. End-stage lung disease: CT findings in 61 patients. *Radiology.* 1993 Dec;189(3): 681-686.

History

▶ 44-year-old woman with chronic shortness of breath and a history of mixed connective tissue disease.

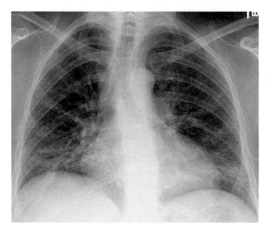

Figure 101.1

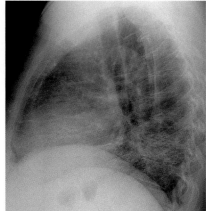

Figure 101.2

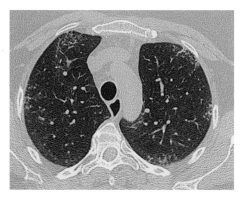

Figure 101.3

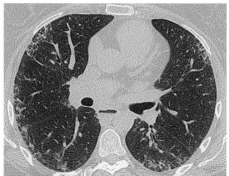

Figure 101.4

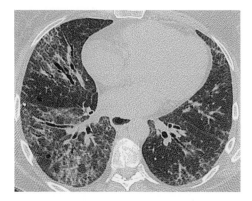

Figure 101.5

Case 101　Nonspecific Interstitial Pneumonia (NSIP)

Figure 101.6

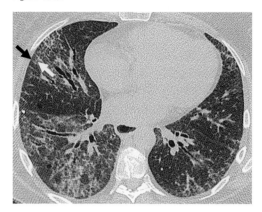

Findings

- Chest radiograph shows coarse linear opacities bilaterally, more confluent in the lower lobes with decreased lung volumes.
- HRCT shows irregular interlobular septal line thickening (black arrow in Fig. 101.6), irregular intralobular septal line thickening (white arrow in Fig. 101.6), traction bronchiectasis, and patchy ground-glass opacities. The combination of interlobular and intralobular septal line thickening is known as reticulation.
- The findings mostly involve the peripheral lung, with gradual increased severity from the apex towards the bases.

Differential Diagnosis

- The differential diagnosis for reticulation with traction bronchiectasis and ground glass with a basilar and peripheral predominance would be led by fibrosis. Given the paucity of honeycombing, nonspecific interstitial pneumonitis (NSIP) should be favored over usual interstitial pneumonitis (UIP). Given the predominance of reticulation over ground glass, NSIP should be favored over desquamative interstitial pneumonitis (DIP).

Teaching Points

- When NSIP is suspected, an underlying cause should be sought. There is a very high association with collagen vascular disease, especially scleroderma, polymyositis, or dermatomyositis. Drugs, occupational exposure, and hypersensitivity pneumonitis are other causes of NSIP.
- Onset is gradual and the symptoms are nonspecific, usually cough and dyspnea on exertion.
- Compared to UIP, NSIP has a better survival rate and prognosis.
- HRCT imaging findings include reticulation, with varying degrees of ground-glass opacities and very little or no honeycombing.
- NSIP tends to be bilateral and symmetric and to favor the lower and peripheral lungs. Atypical findings include centrilobular involvement, subpleural sparing, and uniform diffuse disease.
- Other findings suggestive of connective tissue disease may be seen, including pleural or pericardial effusions, lymphadenopathy, dilated esophagus, basilar bronchiectasis out of proportion to the fibrosis from concomitant aspiration, soft tissue calcification, and joint disease.

Management

- Most cases are treated medically. Lung transplantation is reserved for severe cases refractory to medical treatment.

Further Reading

Jeong YJ, Lee KS, Müller NL, et al. Usual interstitial pneumonia and non-specific interstitial pneumonia: serial thin-section CT findings correlated with pulmonary function. *Korean J Radiol.* 2005 Jul-Sep;6(3):143-152.

Kligerman SJ, Groshong S, Brown KK, et al. Nonspecific interstitial pneumonia: radiologic, clinical, and pathologic considerations. *Radiographics.* 2009 Jan-Feb;29(1):73-87.

History

▸ 71-year-old woman with adenocarcinoma of the lung presents with dyspnea on exertion and increasing cough.

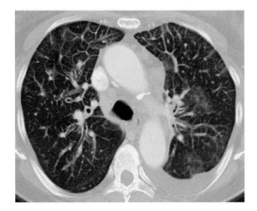

Figure 102.1

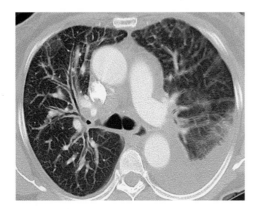

Figure 102.2

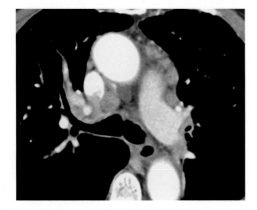

Figure 102.3

Case 102 Lymphangitic Carcinomatosis with Smooth Septal Line Thickening

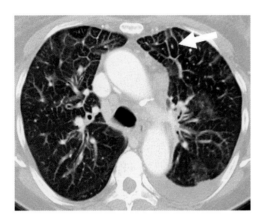

Figure 102.4

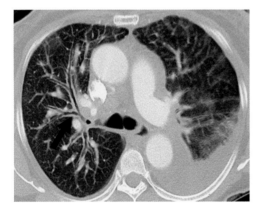

Figure 102.5

Findings

▶ Smooth thickening of the interlobular septa creates polygons anteriorly and bilaterally (arrow in Fig. 102.4). These polygons are the secondary pulmonary lobules.

▶ Smooth peribronchovascular thickening, without associated bronchiectasis can also be seen (black arrow in Fig. 102.5) accompanied by a left pleural effusion and mediastinal lymphadenopathy.

Differential Diagnosis

▶ The main differential diagnosis for smooth septal line thickening is pulmonary edema, especially due to congestive heart failure, or lymphangitic carcinomatosis (LC). A history of malignancy might suggest the latter, but the key to diagnosis rests on the acuity of the pulmonary findings.

Teaching Points

▶ LC represents metastasis to the pulmonary lymphatic system.

▶ LC can result from hematogenous spread to the lymphatics, but much more frequently results from direct invasion of the interstitium and lymphatics.

- Although any tumor can present with LC, it is much more common with adenocarcinomas (especially lung, breast, stomach, pancreas, or colon).
- Patients with LC are usually profoundly symptomatic.
- CT findings consist of smooth or beaded thickening of the peribronchovascular interstitium, smooth or nodular thickening of the interlobular septa, and thickening of the bronchovascular bundle. Any of these features can occur alone.
- LC is focal, unilateral, or asymmetric in approximately 50% of patients. Unilateral LC is much more commonly seen in lung cancer than with other tumors.
- Other common findings are malignant pleural effusions, mediastinal or hilar lymphadenopathy, and pulmonary nodules.
- If ventilation-perfusion scintigraphy is performed, one may find multiple tiny peripheral perfusion defects that accentuate the divisions between lobes and segments (known as segmental contouring or contour mapping).
- Diffuse LC may result in increased lung uptake of FDG on PET.

Management

- LC is a sign of advanced metastatic disease. The patient is usually managed with supportive care.

Further Reading

Johkoh T, Ikezoe J, Tomiyama N, et al. CT findings in lymphangitic carcinomatosis of the lung: correlation with histologic findings and pulmonary function tests. *AJR Am J Roentgenol.* 1992 Jun;158(6):1217-1222.

Schaefer-Prokop C, Prokop M, et al. High-resolution CT of diffuse interstitial lung disease: key findings in common disorders. *Eur Radiol.* 2001;11(3):373-392.

History

▶ 38-year-old woman with history of undifferentiated connective tissue disease has developed progressive dyspnea on exertion and dry cough.

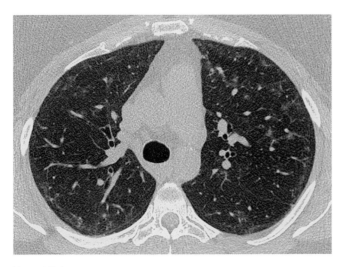

Figure 103.1

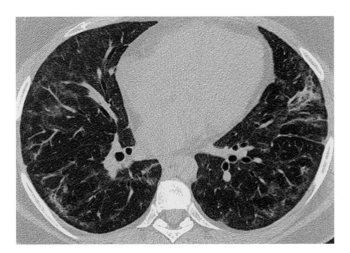

Figure 103.2

Case 103   Desquamative Interstitial Pneumonitis (DIP)

Figure 103.3

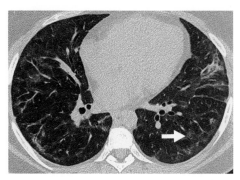

Findings

▸ CT demonstrates multiple patchy areas of ground-glass opacification, favoring the periphery of the lungs and lung bases without reticulation.

Differential Diagnosis

▸ The differential diagnosis based on basilar and peripheral predominant ground-glass opacities includes desquamative interstitial pneumonitis (DIP), organizing pneumonia (OP), and nonspecific interstitial pneumonitis (NSIP). Given the predominance of ground glass over reticulation, DIP or OP should be favored. Although DIP is more common in the bases, OP does not have a zonal predilection.

Teaching Points

▸ DIP accounts for <3% of interstitial pneumonia cases. 90% of those affected are smokers, approximately 30 to 40 years of age.

▸ In never-smokers DIP may be caused by drugs, such as nitrofurantoin, busulphan, and sulfasalazine, connective tissue disease, or dust inhalation.

▸ The term *DIP* is a misnomer based on the incorrect original thought that the cells in the alveolar spaces were desquamated type 2 pneumocytes. In fact, these cells are macrophages, which have been stimulated to aggregate in the alveoli by a trigger, usually cigarette smoke.

▸ Respiratory bronchiolitis interstitial lung disease (RB-ILD) differs from DIP in that the macrophages only have a bronchocentric distribution (centrilobular nodules) and do not fill the alveoli. RB-ILD is also usually upper lobe predominant.

▸ The clinical onset is insidious, presenting as gradually progressive dyspnea and cough.

▸ The most common CT finding is diffuse, patchy, and bilateral ground-glass opacities that favor the lower lungs. About 50% of cases have a subpleural or peripheral distribution. Rarely, cysts may be seen. Architectural distortion is usually mild. Interlobular septal thickening and consolidative opacities are uncommon.

Management

▸ Smoking cessation and oral corticosteroids are the mainstays of therapy. Most patients show significant symptomatic improvement and resolution of ground-glass opacification after a median interval of 11 months of therapy.

▸ In 25% of patients the disease persists or progresses despite therapy.

▸ Progressive disease despite treatment may occur, especially with continued cigarette smoking.

Further Reading

Hansell DM, Nicholson AG. Smoking-related diffuse parenchymal lung disease: HRCT-pathologic correlation. *Semin Respir Crit Care Med.* 2003 Aug;24(4):377-392.

Hidalgo A, Franquet T, Giménez A, et al. Smoking-related interstitial lung diseases: radiologic-pathologic correlation. *Eur Radiol.* 2006 Nov;16(11):2463-2470.

History

▶ 31-year-old man with AIDS (CD4 cell count of 139 cells/microliter) presents with progressive shortness of breath, fever, and dyspnea.

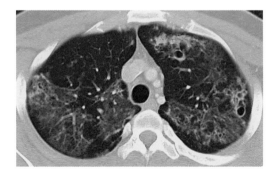

Figure 104.1

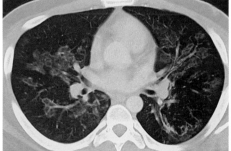

Figure 104.2

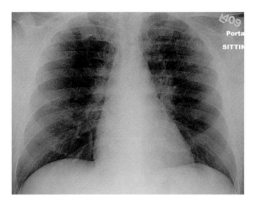

Figure 104.3

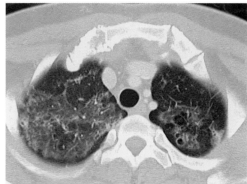

Figure 104.4

Case 104 *Pneumocystis jiroveci* Pneumonia (PCP)

Figure 104.5

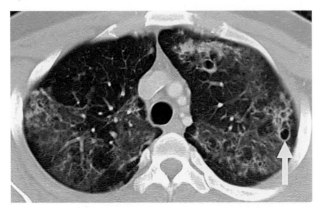

Findings

▸ Portable radiograph (Fig. 104.1) shows very subtle upper-lung-predominant reticulonodular opacities.
▸ CT images confirm the presence of mostly ground-glass opacities with pneumatocele formation (arrow in Fig. 104.5). Pleural effusions and lymphadenopathy are absent.

Differential Diagnosis

▸ The differential diagnosis for ground-glass opacities can be quite long, but when the ground glass is acute, one should consider pneumonia, hemorrhage, or edema (both cardiogenic and noncardiogenic). In patients with HIV, it is important to consider the CD4 cell count. PCP should not be considered when the CD4 count exceeds 200. The absence of effusions and the presence of cysts should favor PCP.

Teaching Points

▸ *Pneumocystis jiroveci* is a unicellular organism that is now considered a fungus.
▸ It is a ubiquitous organism, and infection is believed to represent reactivation in an immunocompromised patient—usually HIV-positive patients with CD4 cell counts <200 who are not on antibiotic prophylaxis. Transplant patients and those who are chronically maintained on corticosteroids are also at risk.
▸ PCP typically presents with a hilar-based symmetric ground-glass pattern. This is always seen on CT but may be missed in up to 10% of chest radiographs, accounting for the reputation of PCP as a radiographically occult pneumonia.
▸ Effusions and lymphadenopathy are typically absent.
▸ CT may show the presence of well-defined cysts (pneumatoceles), which increases the risk of spontaneous pneumothorax (a well-known presenting complaint of patients with PCP).
▸ Rarely, PCP may present with tiny nodules, indicative of a granulomatous variant.

Management

▸ Diagnosis is based on demonstrating the presence of the organism in the sputum. Occasionally, bronchoalveolar lavage is performed to confirm the diagnosis.
▸ Patients with PCP pneumonia should be treated with antibiotics (usually trimethroprim/sulfamethoxazole). Improvement is seen in a few days. In severe cases, patients may require mechanical ventilation.

Further Reading
Bierry G, Boileau J, Barnig C, et al. Thoracic manifestations of primary humoral immunodeficiency: a comprehensive review. *Radiographics.* 2009 Nov;29(7):1909-1920.
Castañer E, Gallardo X, Mata JM, Esteba L. Radiologic approach to the diagnosis of infectious pulmonary diseases in patients infected with the human immunodeficiency virus. *Eur J Radiol.* 2004 Aug;51(2):114-129.

Case 105

History

▶ 78-year-old woman presents with progressive dyspnea.

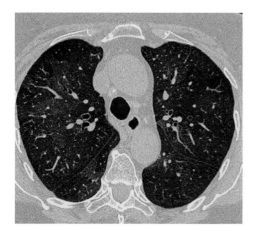

Figure 105.1a

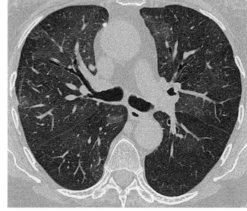

Figure 105.1b

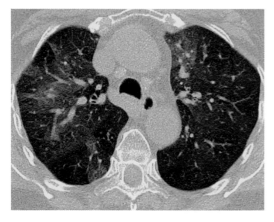

Figure 105.2a

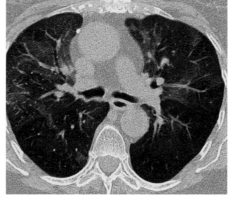

Figure 105.2b

Case 105 Bronchiolitis Obliterans (Constrictive Bronchiolitis)

Findings

▶ HRCT images in inspiration (Fig. 105.1) show mosaic attenuation. Patchy areas of darker lung are associated with attenuated vessels, suggesting that the darker areas are abnormal.

▶ On expiration images (Fig. 105.2), the normal lung becomes more opaque, accentuating the darker areas, indicative of air-trapping.

Differential Diagnosis

▶ Small airways diseases (bronchiolitis obliterans [BO], severe asthma) are favored over small vessels diseases because of air-trapping. Small vessels diseases that may result in mosaic attenuation include chronic pulmonary thromboembolism and vasculitis, but these should not cause air-trapping.

Teaching Points

▶ BO or constrictive bronchiolitis refers to irreversible fibrosis of the small airway walls, resulting in complete replacement of the small airways by scars.

▶ Patients present with obstructive lung disease, progressive dyspnea, and cough.

▶ BO is irreversible and does not respond to corticosteroid treatment.

▶ BO represents a form of chronic rejection in patients who have undergone lung transplantation. Even today, it represents the major cause of long-term mortality in lung transplant recipients.

▶ BO may represent a manifestation of graft-versus-host disease in patients after bone marrow transplantation.

▶ Other potential etiologies of BO include drugs, prior viral infections, collagen vascular disease, toxic inhalation, and inhalation of concentrated flavoring agents (as in microwave popcorn workers). Occasionally, no etiology is discovered.

▶ CT diagnosis of BO is based on HRCT findings of mosaic attenuation with areas of air-trapping. Occasionally, mildly dilated airways and bronchiolar thickening may be seen in the affected areas.

▶ Because of the patchy nature of BO, diagnosis by bronchoscopy can be very difficult. Open lung biopsy is not feasible in the regular follow-up of lung transplant patients. As a result, the term *bronchiolitis obliterans syndrome* (BOS) has been coined to denote those patients in whom a decline in the FEV1 is noted but a histologic diagnosis of BO has not been made.

Management

▶ In post-transplant patients, treatment is aimed at preventing the progression of BO.

▶ In idiopathic BO, treatment is often based on relieving symptoms. The disease does not reverse with medication. Occasionally, patients go on to lung transplantation.

Further Reading

Devakonda A, Raoof S, Sung A, et al. Bronchiolar disorders: a clinical-radiological diagnostic algorithm. *Chest.* 2010;137(4):938-951.

History

▶ 34-year-old man with a long history of obstructive lung disease with acute shortness of breath presents for a two-view chest radiograph.

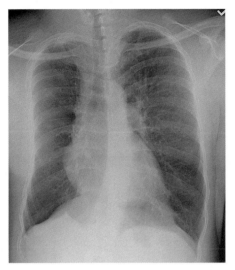

Figure 106.1

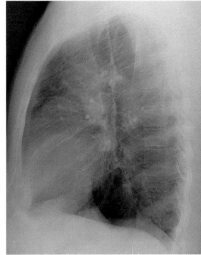

Figure 106.2

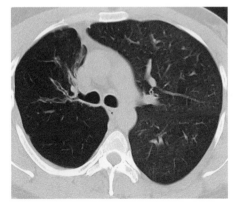

Figure 106.3

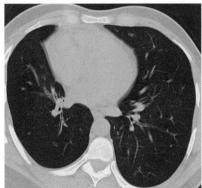

Figure 106.4

Case 106   Swyer-James-Macleod Syndrome (Unilateral Bronchiolitis Obliterans)

Findings

▶ Chest radiograph performed in end-inspiration (Figs. 106.1 and 106.2) shows a smaller right lung with shift of the mediastinum rightward and smaller intercostal spaces. The right lung is also more lucent with attenuated pulmonary vascularity.

▶ CT images (Figs. 106.3 and 106.4) confirm the radiographic findings but also show some mild bronchiectasis in the right lung.

Differential Diagnosis

▶ Based on the hyperlucent lung with volume loss, the differential includes unilateral lung transplant, pulmonary hypoplasia, and Swyer-James-Macleod syndrome.

Teaching Points

▶ Swyer-James-Macleod refers to predominantly unilateral bronchiolitis obliterans, resulting from prior viral or mycoplasma infection.

▶ On chest radiographs, it will present with a smaller, hyperlucent lung that demonstrates air-trapping on expiration images.

▶ The visualization of a smaller lung is key in distinguishing this entity from other causes of unilateral hyperlucent lung such as Poland syndrome (where the lucent lung is normal in size) or congenital lobar overinflation/emphysema (where the lucent lung is larger).

▶ Unlike pulmonary hypoplasia, the vessels are present in Swyer-James-Macleod syndrome, but they are attenuated.

▶ On CT, features of bronchiolitis obliterans will be seen with a smaller, more lucent lung with attenuated vessels. Bronchiectasis may be seen. Areas of bronchiolitis obliterans are usually seen in the contralateral lung as well.

▶ On ventilation-perfusion scintigraphy, the affected lung will show markedly reduced or absent perfusion with retention on the washout ventilation images.

Management

▶ Most patients with Swyer-James-Macleod syndrome will be asymptomatic. However, if the bronchiolitis obliterans is severe enough on the opposite side, patients may have symptoms reflective of their small airways disease (akin to asthma). In this case, the patient had frequent exacerbations of dyspnea related to his bronchiolitis.

Further Reading

Hartman TE, Primack SL, Lee KS, et al. CT of bronchial and bronchiolar diseases. *Radiographics,* 1994;14:991-1003.

Zylak CJ, Eyler WR, Spizarny DL, Stone CH. Developmental lung anomalies in the adult: radiologic-pathologic correlation. *Radiographics.* 2002;22:S25-S43.

History

▸ 42-year-old woman with progressive exertional dyspnea is referred for CT.

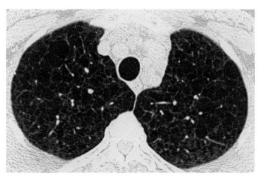

Figure 107.1

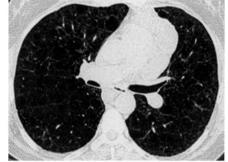

Figure 107.2

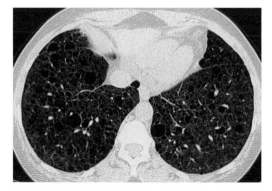

Figure 107.3

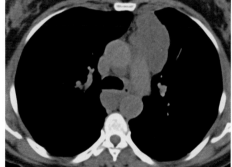

Figure 107.4

Case 107　Lymphangioleiomyomatosis (LAM) (with Mediastinal Lymphangiomas)

Figure 107.5

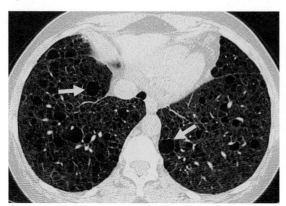

Figure 107.6

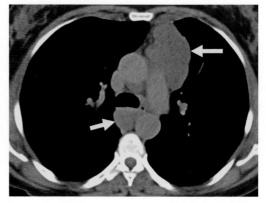

Findings

▶ Diffuse replacement of the lung parenchyma with thin-walled cysts is seen. These cysts can be distinguished from emphysema by the presence of perceptible walls (arrows in Fig. 107.5). Lobular, low-attenuation masses (arrows in Fig. 107.6) are seen in the anterior mediastinum and retrotracheal region, which measure fluid in attenuation.

Differential Diagnosis

▶ The differential is centered on the cystic parenchymal change and includes lymphangioleiomyomatosis (LAM) and Langerhans cell histiocytosis (LCH).

Teaching Points

▶ LAM is a disorder of abnormal proliferation of atypical smooth muscle cells in the lymphatic channels in the pulmonary interstitium and systemic lymphatics.
▶ Cysts in LAM are thought to reflect obstruction of distal airways by abnormal smooth muscle cell proliferation.
▶ On CT, patients with LAM present with round thin-walled cysts of varying size involving the lungs diffusely, including the costophrenic angles. Pulmonary nodules, which can be seen in LCH, are absent.
▶ Usually affecting women of child-bearing age, patients often present with spontaneous pneumothorax or chylous pleural effusions as a result of thoracic duct obstruction.
▶ Mediastinal or abdominal fluid-attenuation masses can develop, reflecting lymphangiomas, which should not be mistaken for lymphadenopathy as can be seen in lymphoma or metastatic disease. Angiomyolipomas can also develop in the kidneys.
▶ LAM can also be seen in the setting of tuberous sclerosis.

Management

▶ Characteristic high-resolution CT findings in the appropriate clinical setting are considered diagnostic. If there is clinical discordance, open lung biopsy establishes the diagnosis.
▶ Supportive treatment is given with lung transplantation for those cases with progressive disease and debilitation. Note should be made that LAM has been reported to recur in a small percentage of lung allografts.

Further Reading

Cosgrove GP, Frankel SK, Brown KK. Challenges in pulmonary fibrosis: cystic lung disease. *Thorax.* 2007 Sep;62(9):820-829.
Lee KH, Lee JS, Lynch DA, et al. The radiologic differential diagnosis of diffuse lung diseases characterized by multiple cysts or cavities. *J Comput Assist Tomogr.* 2002 Jan-Feb;26(1):5-12.

History

▶ 26-year-old smoker with progressive shortness of breath over 6 months.

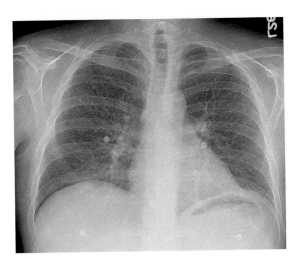

Figure 108.1

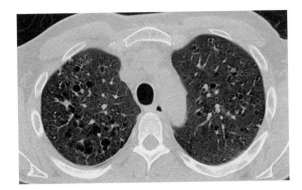

Figure 108.2

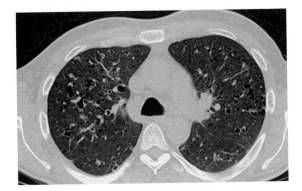

Figure 108.3

Case 108   Langerhans Cell Histiocytosis (Eosinophilic Granuloma [EG])

Figure 108.4

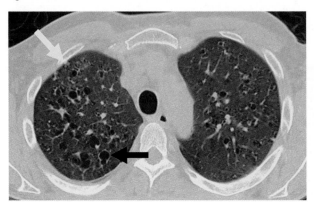

Figure 108.5

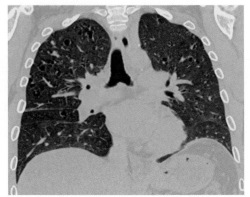

Findings

▸ Chest radiograph (Fig. 108.1) demonstrates upper lobe reticulonodular opacities with preservation of lung volumes.
▸ CT images show tiny nodules (white arrow in Fig. 108.4) and cysts with well-defined walls (black arrow in Fig. 108.4). These upper-lobe-predominant cysts vary in shapes and sizes (Fig. 108.5).

Differential Diagnosis

▸ The differential diagnosis for upper-lobe-predominant cystic areas includes Langerhans cell histiocytosis (LCH), lymphangioleiomyomatosis (LAM), and centrilobular emphysema. The presence of well-defined walls and lack of visualization of a central arteriole would make emphysema unlikely. The heterogeneity of the cysts, the upper lobe predilection and the history of smoking would favor LCH over LAM.

Teaching Points

▸ LCH refers to an idiopathic accumulation of granulomas rich in Langerhans cells and eosinophils. Though many organs may be affected by LCH, isolated pulmonary involvement is well known, occurring in about 40% of all cases.
▸ In adults, >90% of pulmonary LCH cases are observed in patients with a substantial smoking history.
▸ Initially, the granulomas appear as nodules with a perilymphatic pattern. Eventually, the pulmonary destruction results in bizarre-shaped cysts and fibrosis with an upper lung predominance.
▸ LCH can be differentiated from LAM on HRCT by the presence of nodules associated with the cysts and the upper lobe predominance. The cysts in LCH will be irregular in size, shape, and distribution, whereas LAM will have uniform cysts. Also, pleural effusions are quite rare in LCH.
▸ Often LCH may present as a thick-walled cyst ("Cheerio"). The differential for Cheerios would also include bronchioloalveolar carcinoma, Wegener's granulomatosis, or cystic metastatic disease.

Management

▸ Symptoms and findings may regress with smoking cessation.
▸ If the findings are not classic (upper-lobe-predominant cysts with nodules), lung biopsy may be necessary.
▸ Symptomatic patients may require medical therapy. Rarely, patients failing to respond to medical management may go on to lung transplantation.

Further Reading

Abbott GF, Rosado-de-Christenson ML, Franks TJ, et al. From the archives of the AFIP: pulmonary Langerhans cell histiocytosis. *Radiographics*. 2004 May-Jun;24(3):821-841.
Hidalgo A, Franquet T, Giménez A, et al. Smoking-related interstitial lung diseases: radiologic-pathologic correlation. *Eur Radiol*. 2006 Nov;16(11):2463-2470.

History

▶ 24-year-old man with right-sided pleuritic chest pain presents to the Emergency Department.

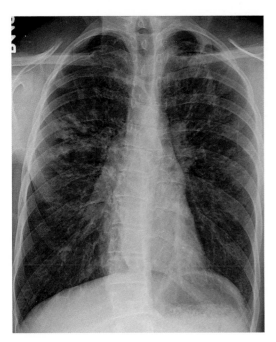

Figure 109.1

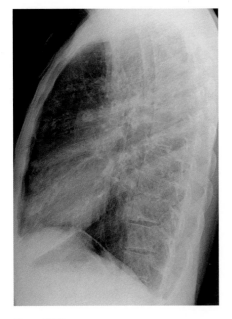

Figure 109.2

Case 109 Cystic Fibrosis

Figure 109.3

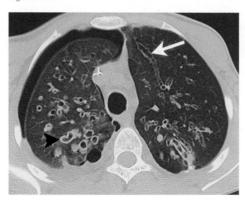

Figure 109.4

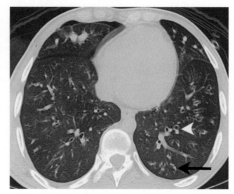

Findings

▶ Chest radiograph (Figs. 109.1 and 109.2) shows increased lung volumes and diffuse interstitial opacities emanating from the hila; many of them are parallel, indicative of bronchiectasis (worse in the upper lungs). Branching tubular densities in the right upper lobe represent mucus impaction in dilated bronchi. A small right pneumothorax is also present.

▶ CT findings include bronchial wall thickening (black arrowhead in Fig. 109.3), tubular and varicoid bronchiectasis (white arrow in Fig. 109.3), signet-ring sign (white arrowhead in Fig. 109.4), mucoid-impacted bronchioles causing tree-in-bud (black arrow in Fig. 109.4), and mosaic attenuation due to air-trapping.

Differential Diagnosis

▶ The causes of bronchiectasis with an upper lobe distribution include cystic fibrosis (CF), allergic bronchopulmonary aspergillosis (more central), and traction bronchiectasis in fibrotic lung disease of the upper lungs.

Teaching Points

▶ CF is an autosomal recessive disease, most commonly seen in white patients.

▶ CF is caused by a mutation in the CF transmembrane conductance regulator that results in dehydration of the endobronchial secretions and poor clearance of the mucus. The net effect is airway obstruction, repeated infections, and subsequent bronchiectasis.

▶ The bronchiectasis can be cylindrical, varicoid, or cystic. It is usually upper lobe predominant.

▶ The signet-ring sign is caused by viewing the dilated, thick-walled bronchus with the adjacent pulmonary artery on cross-section.

▶ The pancreatic ducts can also be affected, leading to pancreatic insufficiency and diabetes mellitus. It is manifested on CT as fat-attenuation parenchyma.

▶ Patients usually present in childhood with variable severity of disease. Cough with sputum production is quite common. Spontaneous pneumothorax and hemoptysis are other frequent clinical presentations.

▶ An abnormal sweat chloride test is diagnostic.

Management

▶ Pulmonary failure accounts for 95% of the deaths. Many patients receive pancreatic enzymes, bronchodilators, prophylactic antibiotics, and aerosolized medications. Bilateral lung transplantation is considered for progressive disease.

Further Reading

Brody AS, Klein JS, Molina PL, et al. High-resolution computed tomography in young patients with cystic fibrosis: distribution of abnormalities and correlation with pulmonary function tests. *J Pediatr.* 2004 Jul;145(1):32-38.

Javidan-Nejad C, Bhalla S. Bronchiectasis. *Thorac Surg Clin.* 2010 Feb;20(1):85-102.

History

▶ 66-year-old man reveals a history of infertility, repeated sinus infections, and pneumonia.

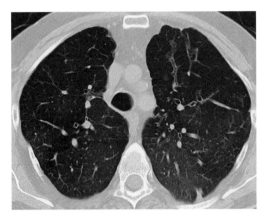

Figure 110.1

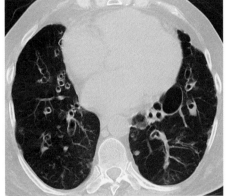

Figure 110.2

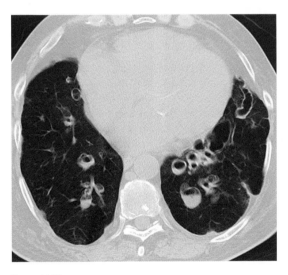

Figure 110.3

Case 110   Immotile Cilia Syndrome or Primary Ciliary Dyskinesia (PCD)

Findings

▶ CT shows bronchial dilatation, wall thickening, and mosaic attenuation. The bronchiectasis is cylindrical in the upper lungs, where the disease is less severe (Fig. 110.1).

▶ Varicoid bronchiectasis in the right middle lobe with mucus impaction in the superior segment of the left lower lobe represents more severe disease (Fig. 110.2).

▶ The basilar segments are the most affected, with cystic bronchiectasis containing air-fluid levels (Fig. 110.3).

Differential Diagnosis

▶ Bronchiectasis with a predilection to the lower lungs can be seen in recurrent infections and conditions that predispose such as chronic aspiration, primary ciliary dyskinesia (PCD), hypogammaglobulinemia, and tracheobronchomegaly (Mounier-Kuhn). Traction bronchiectasis associated with pulmonary fibrosis may also result in lower-lobe-predominant bronchiectasis.

Teaching Points

▶ PCD is an autosomally recessive disease that equally affects men and women.

▶ The defective dynein protein in the cilia leads to abnormal mucociliary function, resulting in mucus retention, repeated pneumonia, bronchiectasis, rhinosinusitis, and otitis media. Affected men are infertile due to immotile spermatozoa. Dyskinetic ciliary activity in the fallopian tubes may contribute to infertility in women.

▶ Kartagener syndrome is a subtype of PCD where there is a triad of situs inversus with dextrocardia, bronchiectasis, and sinusitis.

▶ Morbidity is related to chronic airway infection.

▶ Progression of disease in PCD is slower than in cystic fibrosis.

▶ Diagnosis is made by electron microscopy analysis of the nasal or airway mucosa.

▶ Young syndrome is a rare disease of unknown cause, also associated with repeated sinusitis, bronchiectasis, and infertility. It resembles PCD clinically, but it is not associated with any ciliary abnormality. The azoospermia is caused by inspissated mucus obstructing the epididymis.

▶ Rarely, severe inhalation injury (as in a house fire) may result in lower lobe predominant bronchiectasis, presumably from heat or chemical damage to the mucociliary apparatus.

Management

▶ Prophylactic antibiotics to prevent pseudomonal colonization of the airways are frequently used.

▶ In severe cases, the patients are listed for lung transplantation.

Further Reading

Kennedy MP, Noone PG, Leigh MW, et al. High-resolution CT of patients with primary ciliary dyskinesia. *AJR Am J Roentgenol.* 2007 May;188(5):1232-1238.

History

▶ 54-year-old woman with asthma undergoes radiography and then CT.

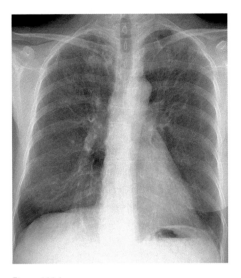

Figure 111.1

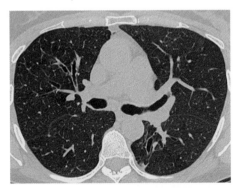

Figure 111.2

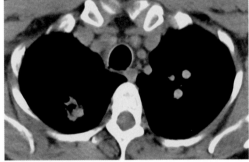

Figure 111.3

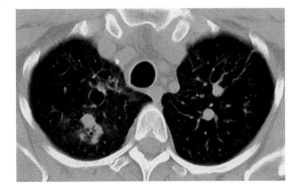

Figure 111.4

Case 111 Allergic Bronchopulmonary Aspergillosis (ABPA)

Figure 111.5

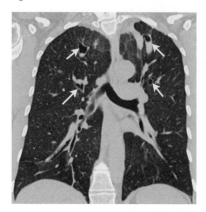

Findings

▸ Chest radiograph (Fig. 111.1) shows tubular lucencies adjacent to both hila and linear densities in bilateral upper lobes.

▸ CT demonstrates bronchiectasis that involves the segmental bronchi and their proximal branches and does not extend to the periphery of the lungs (Fig. 111.2). The bronchiectasis is more severe in the upper lobes (Figs. 111.3 and 111.4).

▸ The apical dilated bronchi are filled with high-density material (Fig. 111.3). Coronal reformation shows the central distribution of the bronchiectasis and with a slight predilection to upper lobes (arrows in Fig. 111.5).

Differential Diagnosis

▸ Both cystic fibrosis and ABPA can cause mucoid impaction and bronchiectasis that favors the upper lobes. The bronchiectasis of ABPA is central, but that of cystic fibrosis is diffuse, extending to the peripheral bronchi and bronchioles.

Teaching Points

▸ The finger-in-glove sign refers to a tubular or branching opacity that radiates from the hilum. It is caused by mucoid impaction of the dilated central bronchi and is seen in many cases of ABPA, including this one.

▸ ABPA is typically seen in patients with chronic asthma and is caused by a hypersensitivity reaction to aspergillus antigens colonizing the airways.

▸ Patients typically present with wheezing, pleuritic chest pain, fever, and expectoration of brown plugs of mucus. Allergic fungal sinusitis may occur with ABPA.

▸ Pathologically, in the dilated bronchi and bronchioles, fungal hyphae without tissue invasion are seen. These are associated with mucoid impaction.

▸ CT features include central bronchiectasis presenting with mucoid impaction, which can occasionally be high in attenuation due to calcium and metallic salts.

▸ Tree-in-bud opacities, air-trapping causing mosaic perfusion, atelectasis, and consolidation are other CT findings.

▸ Diagnosis is established by demonstrating a total serum IgE >500 IU/mL, cutaneous hypersensitivity to aspergillus, or in vitro IgE antibody to aspergillus, in the setting of acute or subacute clinical deterioration with no other cause.

Management

▸ Oral corticosteroid is the treatment of choice.

▸ The response to treatment is monitored by serial measurements of serum IgE.

Further Reading

Martinez S, Heyneman LE, McAdams HP, et al. Mucoid impactions: finger-in-glove sign and other CT and radiographic features. *Radiographics*. 2008 Sep-Oct; 28(5):1369-1382.

History

▶ 76-year-old man with dyspnea has a history of performing boiler insulation in the Navy.

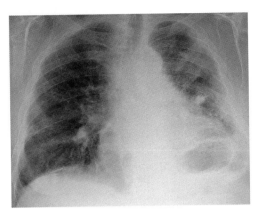

Figure 112.1

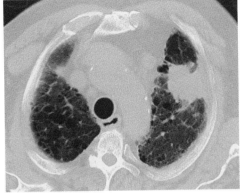

Figure 112.2

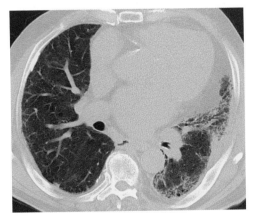

Figure 112.3

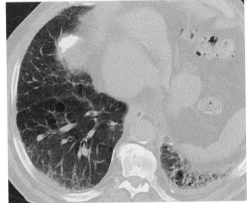

Figure 112.4

Case 112 Asbestosis

Findings

▶ Chest radiograph (Fig. 112.1) shows coarse reticulonodular opacities in the periphery of the lungs. Right hemidiaphragm calcified pleural plaque and left upper lobe opacity are also noted.
▶ CT (Figs. 112.2–112.4) demonstrates reticulation, honeycombing, and traction bronchiectasis in the periphery and bases of the lungs.
▶ CT also confirms pleural plaques and the left upper lobe mass, which turned out to be a lung cancer.

Differential Diagnosis

▶ Asbestosis can simulate nonspecific interstitial pneumonia (when mild), and findings are identical to usual interstitial pneumonia (when severe). The presence of bilateral pleural plaques indicates asbestos exposure, making asbestosis most likely.

Teaching Points

▶ Pleural plaques indicate significant asbestos exposure. *Asbestosis* is used when there is pulmonary fibrosis from the asbestos fibers.
▶ Asbestos occurs naturally as a crystal fiber. It is resistant to heat and chemical corrosion.
▶ In the past, asbestos was used in aircraft manufacturing, building insulation, pipe work, and shipbuilding. It was also used in telephone lines, electric wires, and brakes. Spouses of workers were also exposed to asbestos fibers trapped in the clothing.
▶ Asbestos may result in benign pleural effusions, pleural plaques, rounded atelectasis, or fibrosis (asbestosis).
▶ Diagnosis is achieved without biopsy if there is a history of exposure and typical imaging findings. Demonstrating asbestos bodies in bronchoalveolar lavage fluid is highly specific for the diagnosis.
▶ Irregular reticulation in the periphery of the posterior lungs and ground-glass opacities is an early sign of asbestosis and can simulate dependent atelectasis. Prone CT can help confirm its presence.
▶ With more advanced disease, parenchymal bands (subpleural curvilinear opacities parallel to the pleura), honeycombing, and traction bronchiectasis are seen.
▶ Asbestos exposure increases the risk for mesothelioma and lung cancer (about 20 years after initial exposure).

Management

▶ There is no treatment for asbestosis once the diagnosis has been established.
▶ Because of the higher incidence of neoplasm, smoking cessation and surveillance for cancer should be considered.

Further Reading

Chong S, Lee KS, Chung MJ, et al. Pneumoconiosis: comparison of imaging and pathologic findings. *Radiographics.* 2006 Jan-Feb;26(1):59-77.
Silva CI, Müller NL, Neder JA, et al. Asbestos-related disease: progression of parenchymal abnormalities on high-resolution CT. *J Thoracic Imaging.* 2008 Nov;23(4):251-257.

Case 113

History

▶ 62-year-old man (never smoker) complains of chronic cough and dyspnea.

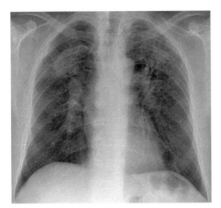

Figure 113.1

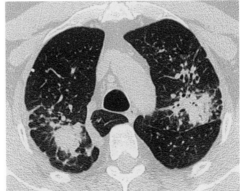

Figure 113.2

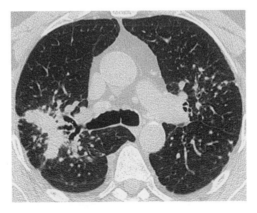

Figure 113.3

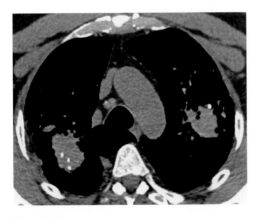

Figure 113.4

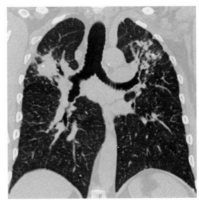

Figure 113.5

293

Case 113   Silicosis

Figure 113.6

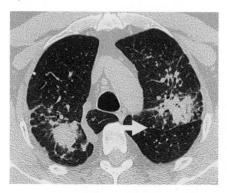

Findings

▶ Chest radiograph (Fig. 113.1) shows mass-like opacities in the upper lungs bilaterally. Reticulonodular opacities surround these masses and volume loss is seen.
▶ CT shows tiny perilymphatic nodules, closely associated with the thickened interlobular septa, pleura, and bronchovascular bundles (Figs. 113.2 and 113.3). Note the beaded fissure (arrow in Fig. 113.6).
▶ Triangular masses with internal punctuate calcification are associated with traction bronchiectasis (Figs. 113.2–113.5).

Differential Diagnosis

▶ The main differential diagnosis of micronodular lung disease with an upper lung distribution and associated conglomerate mass-like fibrosis includes silicosis, coal-worker pneumoconiosis, and sarcoidosis. A history of exposure to silica allows silicosis to be the leading diagnosis.

Teaching Points

▶ *Silicosis* refers to fibrosis caused by inhalation of silica dust.
▶ Diagnosis requires a history of exposure to silica, usually >20 years, and characteristic imaging findings.
▶ Occupations typically providing exposure include mining, sandblasting, quarrying, and tunneling.
▶ Silicosis has two radiographic patterns: simple and complicated.
▶ HRCT of simple silicosis is characterized by well-defined pulmonary nodules, measuring 2 to 5 mm in size, mostly in the posterior upper lobes. The nodules calcify in 10% to 20% of patients and tend to be perilymphatic.
▶ In complicated silicosis, the nodules conglomerate to create areas of mass-like fibrosis (progressive massive fibrosis [PMF]) >1 cm in diameter in the middle and upper lungs. Paracicatricial emphysema between the masses and pleural surface is common. Typically, the lateral margin of the mass parallels the lateral chest wall (Fig. 113.1). PMF usually calcifies and can demonstrate central cavitation.
▶ *Candle wax lesions* refer to visceral pleural nodules that can create pseudo-plaques when confluent.
▶ Eggshell nodal calcification is seen in both silicosis and sarcoidosis.
▶ The risk of tuberculosis and lung cancer is higher in silicosis.
▶ PMF may have intense metabolic activity on FDG-PET due to active fibrosis.

Management

▶ There is no specific treatment for silicosis.

Further Reading

Chong S, Lee KS, Chung MJ, et al. Pneumoconiosis: comparison of imaging and pathologic findings. *Radiographics.* 2006 Jan-Feb; 26(1):59-77.
Marchiori E, Ferriera A, Saez F, et al. Conglomerated masses of silicosis in sandblasters: high-resolution CT findings. *Eur J Rad.* 2006;59:56-59.

History

▶ 41-year-old woman with chronic dyspnea. She also has a history of cholangiocarcinoma, for which she received a liver transplant 9 months prior.

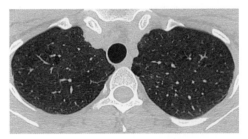

Figure 114.1

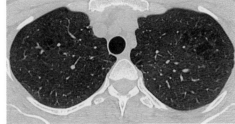

Figure 114.2

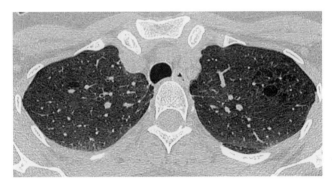

Figure 114.3

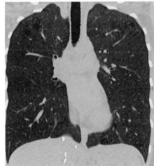

Figure 114.4

Case 114 Centrilobular Emphysema

Figure 114.5

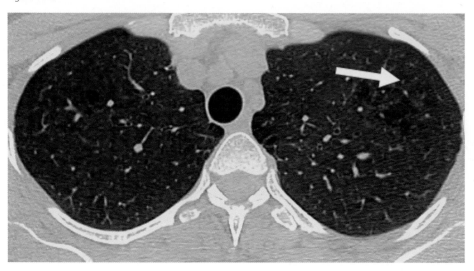

Findings

▶ CT images show upper-lobe-predominant lucent areas without definable walls.
▶ No air-trapping is seen on the expiration image (Fig. 114.3).
▶ Note how the lucencies surround the centrilobular arterioles (arrow in Fig. 114.5).

Differential Diagnosis

▶ Centrilobular emphysema should lead the differential diagnosis. Though one might consider upper lobe cystic lung disease, such as Langerhans cell histiocytosis or pneumatoceles of pneumocystic pneumonia (PCP), the lack of definable walls and the identification of the centrilobular arterioles make these diagnoses highly unlikely.

Teaching Points

▶ Emphysema is classified according to the part of the acinus that is involved. Centrilobular emphysema involves the proximal acinus, while pan-acinar emphysema involves the whole acinus. Paraseptal emphysema involves the distal acinus.
▶ Centrilobular emphysema can be diagnosed by the characteristic lucencies surrounding the centrilobular structures.
▶ Centrilobular emphysema is strongly associated with cigarette smoking.
▶ When it is more severe, the lucent areas may coalesce and the centrilobular arterioles may no longer be seen. Distinction from pan-acinar emphysema, then, becomes more difficult.
▶ Unlike pan-acinar emphysema, centrilobular emphysema has a predilection for the upper lobes.
▶ Paraseptal emphysema tends to be subpleural and is often associated with centrilobular emphysema. It is only rarely seen in isolation.
▶ Centrilobular emphysema tends to be scattered throughout the lung parenchyma. Spared areas of lung may, at times, may be confused for ground-glass opacities.
▶ The lucent areas usually do not have well-defined walls. Rarely, fibrosis around emphysematous regions can simulate a thin wall.

Management

▶ Most patients are mildly symptomatic in the early stages of the disease.

▶ Clinical symptoms will guide the clinician more than imaging. When the disease is severe, patients may require lung transplantation.

▶ In reporting emphysema, the presence of any dominant bulla and extent of disease should be included. If surgery is contemplated, a dominant bulla may prompt a bullectomy. Upper-lobe-dominant disease with spared lower lobes may push the patient to volume-reduction surgery. Severe, diffuse disease without a dominant bulla and little to no normal lung will make lung transplantation the dominant surgical option.

Further Reading

Newell JD Jr. CT of emphysema. *Radiol Clin North Am.* 2002 Jan;40(1):31-42.

History

▶ 52-year-old man with history of dyspnea undergoes routine chest radiography.

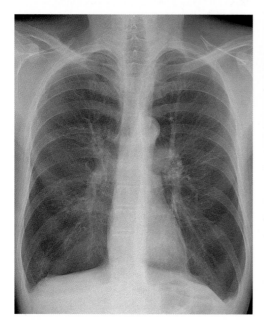

Figure 115.1

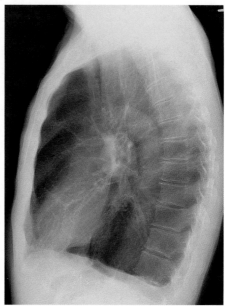

Figure 115.2

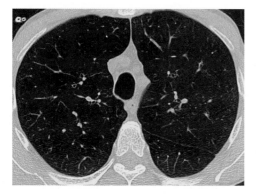

Figure 115.3

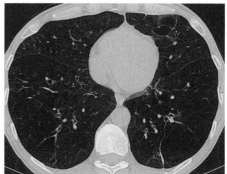

Figure 115.4

Case 115   Alpha-1 Antitrypsin Deficiency with Pan-Lobular (Pan-Acinar) Emphysema

Findings

▶ The chest radiograph show lower-lobe-predominant emphysema with increased lung volumes (Figs. 115.1 and 115.2).
▶ Thin-section CT confirms the radiographic findings (Figs. 115.3 and 115.4), with increased lucency affecting the entire secondary pulmonary lobule. The process is more severe in the bases and is associated with lower lobe bronchiectasis and scarring.

Differential Diagnosis

▶ The differential comprises pan-lobular (pan-acinar) emphysema, centrilobular emphysema, and bronchiolitis obliterans.

Teaching Points

▶ Pan-lobular/pan-acinar emphysema affects the entire secondary lobule uniformly. It can be differentiated from centrilobular emphysema by the lack of visualization of the central arteriole and bronchiole on HRCT.
▶ Pan-lobular emphysema tends to be more severe in the lower lobes. This distribution has been postulated to be related to the increased blood flow and increased number of neutrophils and macrophages (the source of the alpha-1 antiprotease) in the bases.
▶ When mild, pan-acinar emphysema can be hard to separate from bronchiolitis obliterans and other small airways diseases.
▶ Similar pathologic findings can be seen in the emphysema associated with excessive intravenous drug use, most notably methylphenidate (Ritalin).
▶ Alpha-1 antitrypsin deficiency is also associated with bronchial wall thickening and bronchiectasis.
▶ The lung destruction in this condition can be accelerated by cigarette use.
▶ Lower-lobe-predominant emphysema should prompt one to consider alpha-1 antitrypsin deficiency or intravenous drug abuse (most notably Ritalin).
▶ Ventilation-perfusion scintigraphy typically shows increased retention of xenon and decreased perfusion in the lower lobes bilaterally.

Management

▶ Most patients are mildly symptomatic in the early stages of the disease.
▶ Clinical symptoms will guide the clinician more than imaging. When the disease is severe, patients may require lung transplantation.

Further Reading

Newell JD Jr. CT of emphysema. *Radiol Clin North Am.* 2002 Jan;40(1):31-42.

History

▶ 29-year-old man with HIV develops fever and dyspnea during his admission.

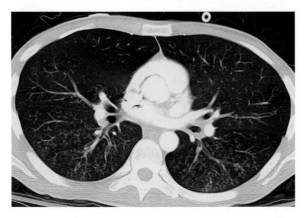

Figure 116.1

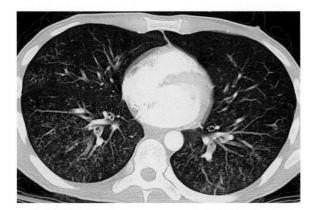

Figure 116.2

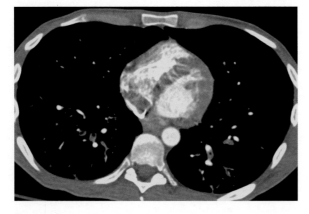

Figure 116.3

Case 116 Aspiration Causing Tree-In-Bud Pattern

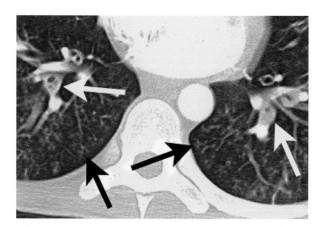

Figure 116.4

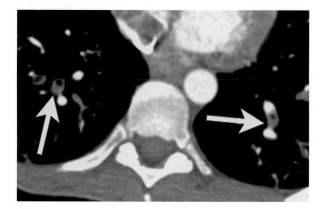

Figure 116.5

Findings

▶ CT images show fine centrilobular nodules with branching structures, creating the appearance of tree-in-bud (TIB) (black arrows on Fig. 116.4). The distribution is mainly in the lower lobes, especially in the posterior basal and lateral segments.

▶ The segmental bronchi are dilated and filled with fluid-density material on the soft-tissue window setting (white arrows in Fig. 116.5).

Differential Diagnosis

▶ The differential diagnosis rests on the pattern of TIB and the location of findings. Although TIB may be seen with aspiration, infectious bronchiolitis (viral infections, tuberculosis, and atypical mycobacterial infection), or bronchiectasis (cystic fibrosis, ciliary dyskinesia, and bronchopulmonary aspergillosis), the distribution in this case would favor aspiration.

Teaching Points

▶ Aspiration causes an inflammatory and infectious bronchitis and bronchiolitis, due to foreign material into the airways. The aspirated material can be food, gastric secretions, blood, or pus.

- Abnormalities of the esophagus can lead to chronic aspiration. These include achalasia, esophageal diverticulum, gastroesophageal reflux disease, scleroderma and other dysmotility diseases, esophageal cancer, and gastric pull-through surgery.
- Neurologic abnormalities, and hospitalization can also predispose to aspiration.
- Chest radiography may be normal or may show reticulonodular opacities in the lower lobes.
- TIB on HRCT is characterized by relatively well-defined centrilobular nodules 1 to 3 mm in size, clustered around end arterioles or dilated bronchioles. They appear as branching nodular opacities.
- TIB typically spares the lung 5 to 10 mm from the pleura and fissures.
- In aspiration, TIB mostly involves the dependent lung.
- Endobronchial mucus and air bubbles are common in acute aspiration. Findings of surrounding pneumonia can be seen.
- Wall thickening and dilatation of the segmental bronchi and bronchioles in the involved portions can be evident with chronic aspiration.

Management

- TIB implies the presence of endobronchial disease. Consequently, diagnosis of a process causing TIB is usually by bronchoscopy. In the case of aspiration, bronchoscopy is usually unnecessary.
- Management is aimed at preventing further bouts of aspiration and treating any concomitant pneumonia.

Further Reading

Rossi SE, Franquet T, Volpacchio M, et al. Tree-in-bud pattern at thin-section CT of the lungs: radiologic-pathologic overview. *Radiographics*. 2005 May-Jun;25(3):789-801.

History

▶ 67-year-old woman (never smoker) complains of persistent shortness of breath and cough.

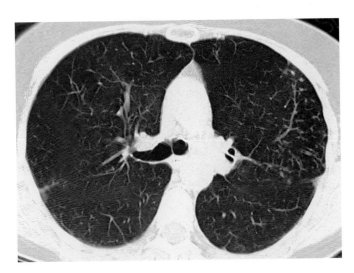

Figure 117.1

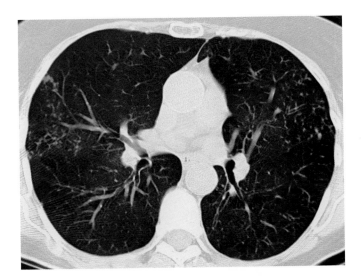

Figure 117.2

Case 117　*Mycobacterium avium complex* (MAC) Pneumonia

Figure 117.3

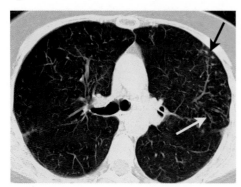

Figure 117.4

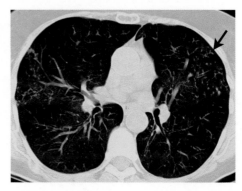

Findings

▶ CT demonstrates 1- to 2-mm nodules in the lingula and right middle lobe. The nodules have a centrilobular distribution and create a tree-in-bud (TIB) pattern (black arrows in Figs. 117.3 and 117.4).

▶ Mildly dilated bronchioles (white arrow in Fig. 117.3) are seen.

Differential Diagnosis

▶ Differential diagnosis is based on a TIB pattern with an upper lobe, middle lobe, and lingular distribution. Mycobacterial infection, aspiration, and endobronchial bronchioloalveolar carcinoma can result in TIB. When combined with the location and the patient's demographic information, mycobacterial infection would be favored.

Teaching Points

▶ Nontuberculous mycobacteria (NTM), unlike *Mycobacterium* tuberculosis (TB), are not obligate human pathogens. They are commonly isolated from the environment, such as soil and fresh water. Human transmission does not occur in immunocompetent hosts, obviating the need for isolation techniques.

▶ In the United States *M. avium complex* (MAC) and *M. kansasii* are the two most common causes of NTM pulmonary disease.

▶ Pulmonary NTM has three different presentations in immunocompetent adults: (1) fibrocavitary pattern in the upper lobes, simulating reactivation TB, seen mostly in elderly men with COPD; (2) nodular bronchiectatic form, mostly involving the right middle lobe and lingula, seen in nonsmoking, slender, older women (Lady Windermere syndrome); and (3) hypersensitivity pneumonitis, acquired with use of hot tubs with colonized water.

▶ Gastroesophageal reflux and chest wall disorders are also predisposing factors.

▶ Chronic productive cough and fatigue are frequent symptoms. Fever and sweats are less common than TB. Weight loss and hemoptysis reflect advanced disease.

▶ Diagnosis is based on a combination of clinical symptoms, imaging findings, and positive microbiology.

▶ As NTM look identical to TB on acid-fast stains and tend to be slowly growing organisms, diagnosis may be made by genetic analysis as opposed to culture.

▶ MAC is distributed mainly in the right middle lobe and lingula. Air-trapping is common.

Management

▶ Treatment is similar to TB, with a three- or four-drug regimen. Sometimes, patients forego treatment, as the drug side effects may be worse than the symptoms.

Further Reading

Glassroth J. Pulmonary disease due to nontuberculous mycobacteria. *Chest.* 2008 Jan;133(1):243-251.

Koh WJ, Kwon OJ, Lee KS. Nontuberculous mycobacterial pulmonary diseases in immunocompetent patients. *Korean J Radiol.* 2002;3(3):145-157.

History

▶ 62-year-old man with asthma complains of worsening cough, fatigue, and shortness of breath over the past 3 to 6 months.

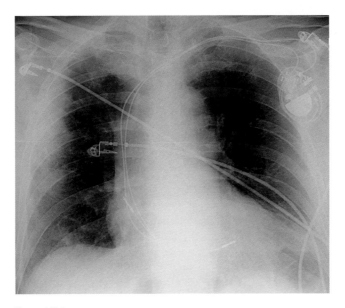

Figure 118.1

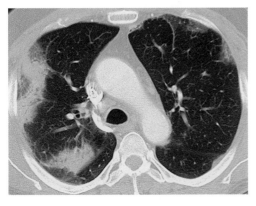

Figure 118.2

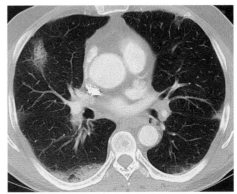

Figure 118.3

Case 118   Chronic Eosinophilic Pneumonia

Figure 118.4

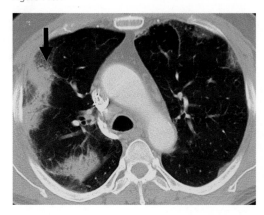

Findings

▶ Chest radiograph (Fig. 118.1) shows mostly peripheral airspace opacities in the right mid-lung and right lung base and to a lesser extent the left mid-lung.

▶ CT confirms the multiple areas of pleural-based consolidations (Figs. 118.2 and 118.3). Many are wedge-shaped. One of the regions of consolidation is less dense close to the pleura (arrow in Fig. 118.4), allowing it to attain a somewhat linear appearance.

Differential Diagnosis

▶ The differential diagnosis for peripheral consolidation consists mainly of pulmonary infarct, organizing pneumonia, and eosinophilic pneumonia (simple eosinophilic pneumonia, chronic eosinophilic pneumonia, and eosinophilic pneumonia with vasculitis [Churg-Strauss syndrome]). Given the time course of this patient's symptoms and lack of other organ involvement, organizing pneumonia (OP) and chronic eosinophilic pneumonia (CEP) would be favored.

Teaching Points

▶ CEP is a chronic, progressive, eosinophilic lung disease.

▶ Diagnosis is suggested by peripheral eosinophilia and confirmed with tissue eosinophilia at lung biopsy, or increased eosinophils in bronchoalveolar lavage fluid.

▶ CEP has an insidious onset, with an average of 7.7 months of fever, weight loss, night sweats, and dyspnea.

▶ 50% of patients with CEP have asthma.

▶ The characteristic appearance consists of bilateral peripheral consolidation in a distribution opposite that seen in severe pulmonary edema, often called the "photographic negative of pulmonary edema."

▶ CEP can be asymmetric. Pleural effusions are rare.

▶ CT often shows homogenous nonsegmental consolidations, which abut the pleura and favor the upper lungs.

▶ On pathology, areas of organizing pneumonia are frequently seen in CEP, which accounts for the overlap in imaging features between CEP and OP.

Management

▶ CEP responds well to oral corticosteroid therapy with a good prognosis. Occasional relapse can be seen, prompting a repeat course of steroids.

Further Reading

Jeong YJ, Kim KI, Seo IJ, et al. Eosinophilic lung diseases: a clinical, radiologic, and pathologic overview. *Radiographics.* 2007;27:617-639.
Sano S, Yamagami K, Yoshioka K. Chronic eosinophilic pneumonia: a case report and review of the literature. *Cases J.* 2009 Jul 2;2:7735.
Silva CI, Colby TV, Müller NL. Asthma and associated conditions: high-resolution CT and pathologic findings. *AJR Am J Roentgenol.* 2004 Sep;183(3):817-824.

Part 13   Pulmonary Vascular Diseases

History

▸ 78-year-old man with high-grade urothelial carcinoma presents with dyspnea.

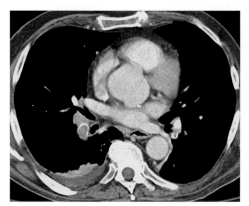

Figure 119.1

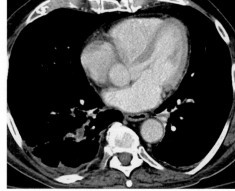

Figure 119.2

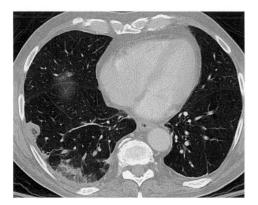

Figure 119.3

Case 119 Acute Pulmonary Embolism with Pulmonary Infarcts

Figure 119.4

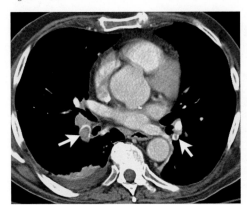

Figure 119.5

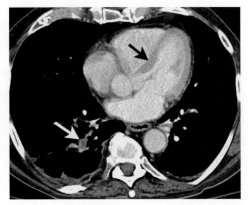

Findings

▶ CTA of the pulmonary arteries shows filling defects (white arrows in Figs. 119.4 and 119.5) in the lower lobe pulmonary arteries. The filling defects expand the arteries (Fig. 119.2).

▶ The interventricular septum is bowed toward the left ventricle (black arrow in Fig. 119.5), suggesting right ventricular strain.

▶ Lung windows reveal peripheral wedge-shaped consolidations and ground-glass opacities (Fig. 119.3).

Differential Diagnosis

▶ Intravascular filling defects of the pulmonary arteries are most commonly due to pulmonary embolism (PE). Other filling defects include sarcoma and tumor emboli. These latter entities may enhance.

Teaching Points

▶ Acute PE is the third most common acute cardiovascular disease, after myocardial infarction and stroke.

▶ The most common underlying factors are immobilization and malignancy.

▶ Symptoms are nonspecific and may include sudden onset of dyspnea, chest pain, tachycardia, and syncope.

▶ D-dimer test has a high sensitivity and poor specificity; it is used to exclude acute PE.

▶ Chest radiography is an unreliable means of diagnosis. Decreased vascularity in the peripheral lung (Westermark sign), enlargement of the central pulmonary artery (Fleischner sign), and pleural-based areas of increased opacity (Hampton sign) are signs of acute PE but are nonspecific.

▶ Pulmonary CTA is now considered the gold standard of diagnosis and may provide alternative diagnoses in negative cases.

▶ On CT an intraluminal filling defect with acute margins relative to the arterial wall is usually seen. Abrupt cutoff of the intraluminal contrast in an expanded vessel may also be seen.

▶ Care must be used to confirm that the filling defect is within an artery and not in a vein or a mucus plug within a bronchus.

▶ Acute PE may be associated with pulmonary infarction. Infarcts appear as wedge-shaped, pleural-based consolidations and do not enhance.

▶ Massive PE can cause right ventricle (RV) strain, which manifests as RV enlargement, without RV hypertrophy.

Management

▶ Anticoagulation is the mainstay of treatment.

▶ Inferior vena cava filters are placed for those at risk of intracranial or gastric hemorrhage.

▶ Thrombolysis and thrombectomy are considered for those with massive PE causing systemic hypotension.

Further Reading

Kuriakose J, Patel S. Acute pulmonary embolism. *Radiol Clin North Am.* 2010 Jan;48(1):31-50.

History

▶ 26-year-old woman with dyspnea is imaged.

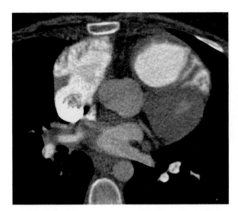

Figure 120.1

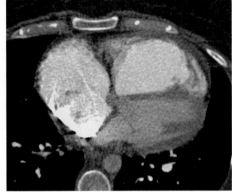

Figure 120.2

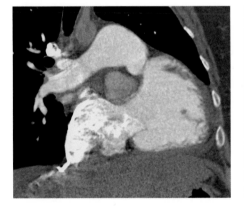

Figure 120.3

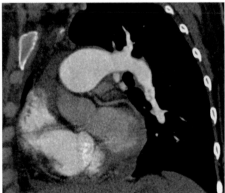

Figure 120.4

Case 120   Chronic Pulmonary Embolism

Figure 120.5

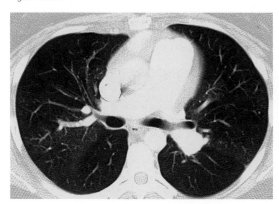

Figure 120.6

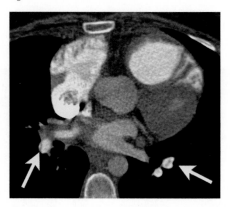

Findings

▶ Pulmonary CTA shows linear filling defects in the pulmonary arteries (arrows in Fig. 120.6). The atrial septum is bowed to the left, the right ventricle is thick-walled, and the interventricular septum is flattened (Fig. 120.2). The main pulmonary artery is enlarged.

▶ Reconstructions show intraluminal linear filling defects with beading and pruning of the affected vessels (Figs. 120.3 and 120.4).

▶ Lung window (Fig. 120.5) shows mosaic attenuation.

Differential Diagnosis

▶ The differential diagnosis for webs within the pulmonary arteries with CT findings of pulmonary hypertension and mosaic attenuation is headed by chronic pulmonary embolism (PE). The webs can be seen with incompletely resolved acute PE, but mosaic attenuation and findings of pulmonary hypertension should not be seen. Vasculitis and small airways disease can present with mosaic attenuation, but intraluminal webs should be absent.

Teaching Points

▶ Chronic PE refers to cytokine-mediated scarring that may follow even one episode of acute PE. In fact, up to 4% of patients with acute PE may go on to chronic PE. It is more than simply an old acute PE.

▶ Risk factors include malignancies, prior splenectomy, chronic inflammatory disorders, and ventriculoatrial shunts.

▶ Clinical symptoms are nonspecific and occur when pulmonary hypertension and right ventricular dysfunction have developed.

▶ The direct signs on CT include tapering of the artery, complete cutoff of the artery, wall thickening with intimal irregularity, and webs or beading of the vessel. Such findings are usually better demonstrated on multiplanar reconstructions or MIPs.

▶ The central pulmonary arteries tend to be enlarged. Cardiac findings include right ventricular hypertrophy, right atrial enlargement, and commonly a patent foramen ovale with right-to-left shunting.

▶ Tortuous and enlarged bronchial collateral arteries and bronchiectasis are also usually present.

Management

▶ Lifelong anticoagulation is recommended to prevent recurrent PE.

▶ Pulmonary thromboendarterectomy is used for more central disease. Patients with more peripheral disease are usually treated for the pulmonary hypertension.

Further Reading

Castañer E, Xavier Gallardo X, Ballesteros E, et al. CT diagnosis of chronic pulmonary thromboembolism. *Radiographics.* 2009;29:31-53.

History

► 73-year-old woman awoke with sudden substernal chest tightness and pressure.

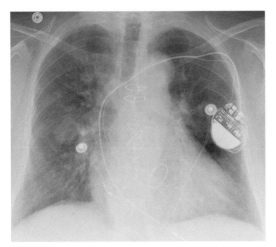

Figure 121.1

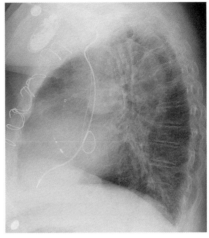

Figure 121.2

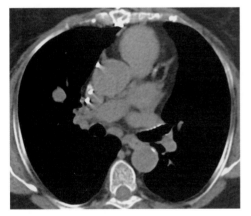

Figure 121.3

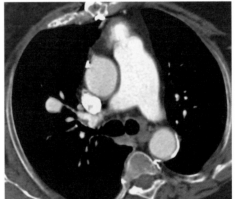

Figure 121.4

Case 121   Pulmonary Artery Pseudoaneurysm

Figure 121.5

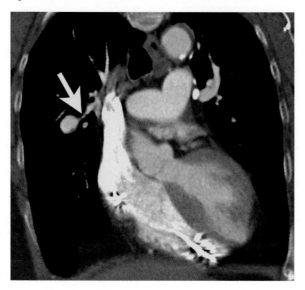

Findings

▶ Chest radiograph shows a well-circumscribed nodule adjacent to the right hilum.
▶ CT (Figs. 121.3 and 121.4) before and after intravenous contrast administration demonstrates uniform enhancement of this nodule, with similar attenuation to the main pulmonary artery.
▶ CT reconstruction (Fig. 121.5) demonstrates a small pulmonary artery connecting to this nodule (arrow).

Differential Diagnosis

▶ The differential diagnosis is based on the presence of a vigorously enhancing nodule with a small arterial feeder. Although pseudoaneurysms (PSAs), aneurysms, varices, arteriovenous malformations, and hypervascular neoplasms (most notably carcinoid) can present with an enhancing nodule, only PSAs and aneurysms will have connection with an artery and no draining vein.

Teaching Points

▶ A pulmonary artery PSA, contrary to a true aneurysm, does not involve all layers of the arterial wall and is at risk of rupture.
▶ Pulmonary PSA is most commonly caused by a contained perforation of the arterial wall after placement of a pulmonary arterial catheter too peripherally.
▶ Other iatrogenic causes include trauma of the artery after stab, gunshot injury, intrapulmonary chest tube placement, or after biopsy or surgery.
▶ Infectious PSAs can be caused by bacteria. These mostly occur in intravenous drug users with infectious endocarditis and septic emboli.
▶ Aggressive local infection, most notably tuberculosis and mucormycosis, can perforate the arterial wall, causing PSAs. The PSA caused by tuberculosis is called a Rasmussen aneurysm.
▶ Malignancies such as lung cancer and metastatic sarcomas may also cause PSAs by eroding into the vessels.

- Patients may give a history of gradually increasing hemoptysis. If iatrogenic, the PSA may be quiescent for a long period of time, only to become symptomatic after sudden rupture.
- CTA reveals an arterial enhancing well-circumscribed nodule, which may have peripheral thrombus and surrounding ground-glass opacities, indicative of some pulmonary hemorrhage. Connection with a pulmonary artery should be seen.

Management

- Coil embolization is the treatment of choice for most of these PSAs. In the setting of infection or severe trauma, lobectomy may be required.

Further Reading

Nguyen ET, Silva CIS, Seely JM, et al. Pulmonary artery aneurysms and pseudoaneurysms in adults: findings at CT and radiography. *AJR Am J Roentgenol.* 2007;188:W126-W134.

History

▶ 34-year-old woman with dyspnea on exertion and recent syncope.

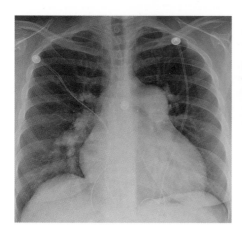

Figure 122.1

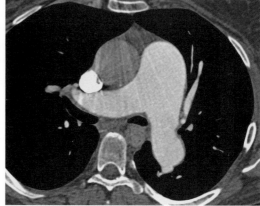

Figure 122.2

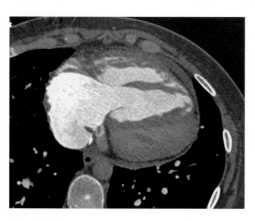

Figure 122.3

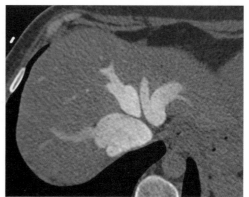

Figure 122.4

Case 122 Pulmonary Hypertension (Idiopathic Pulmonary Arterial Hypertension)

Findings

▶ Chest radiograph shows a large convexity in the region of the aortopulmonary window corresponding to the main pulmonary artery (Fig. 125.1). Note the abrupt change in caliber from enlarged central vessels to peripheral absence, referred to as pruning.

▶ CT shows marked enlargement of pulmonary arteries. The right ventricle (RV) is hypertrophied. The interventricular septum is bowed towards the left ventricle. A small pericardial effusion is seen.

Differential Diagnosis

▶ Enlarged main pulmonary artery (PA) can be seen with pulmonary hypertension (PH), pulmonic stenosis, and a rare entity, idiopathic dilation of the pulmonic trunk. Unlike the latter two entities, PH affects the main and right and left pulmonary arteries and is accompanied by RV hypertrophy.

Teaching Points

▶ The term *pulmonary arterial hypertension* (PAH) is reserved for entities belonging to group 1 of the 2008 World Health Organization Classification in which the pathology resides in the pulmonary arterial walls. These entities include idiopathic PAH, PAH associated with connective tissue disease, portal hypertension, HIV, and congenital heart disease.

▶ The increased vascular resistance in PAH is caused by remodeling of the vessel wall with intimal fibrosis and hyperplasia of the smooth muscle causing vasoconstriction.

▶ PAH has a poor prognosis without treatment. The median life expectancy after diagnosis of idiopathic PAH is 2.8 years.

▶ PH is a more generic term that includes PAH and other entities that elevate PA pressures, including chronic PE, left heart disease, and hypoxic lung disease.

▶ CT features of PH are a cross-sectional diameter of the main PA larger than that of the ascending aorta or >29 mm in adults with RV hypertrophy. Pruning of the PAs is usually a feature of PAH.

▶ MR may be used to follow RV function after treatment has been initiated.

Management

▶ The treatment regimen varies by cause of PH and severity of disease.

▶ Vasodilator therapy has made major inroads for the treatment of PAH, reserving transplant for the few cases that are refractory to medical management.

Further Reading

Grosse C, Grosse A. CT findings in diseases associated with pulmonary hypertension: a current review. *Radiographics*. 2010;30: 1753-1777.

History

▶ 82-year-old woman who had a left mastectomy 40 years ago, who presents to the Emergency Department with a tingling sensation in her chest for 2 weeks.

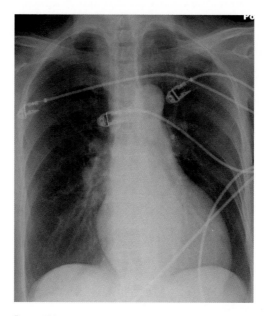

Figure 123.1

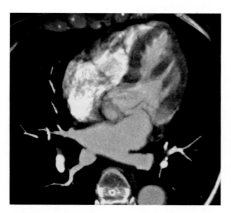

Figure 123.2

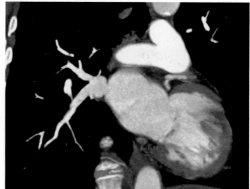

Figure 123.3

Case 123   Pulmonary Vein Varix

Figure 123.4

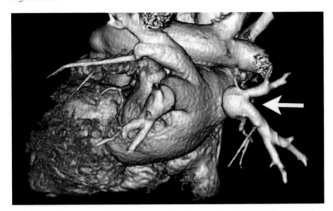

Findings

▶ Chest radiograph (Fig. 123.1) shows a nodular opacity in the right hilum.
▶ Maximum-intensity projection images show nodular dilation of the right inferior pulmonary vein (Figs. 123.2 and 123.3).
▶ Volume-rendered image (Fig. 123.4) demonstrates enlargement of the right inferior pulmonary vein (arrow) relative to the other pulmonary veins.

Differential Diagnosis

▶ The differential diagnosis for a vascular nodule includes a pulmonary varix, arteriovenous malformation, and pulmonary artery aneurysm/pseudoaneurysm. Connecting this to the vein without a feeding artery confirms the diagnosis of varix.

Teaching Points

▶ Pulmonary vein varix (PVV) is an uncommon lesion where a segment of the pulmonary vein is abnormally enlarged.
▶ PVVs are usually asymptomatic and incidental. Because a PVV can simulate a pulmonary nodule on chest radiography, it often leads to diagnostic workup by CT.
▶ PVV is always solitary and in 75% of cases involves the right inferior pulmonary vein.
▶ Most PVVs are congenital. Acquired PVVs are seen with mitral valve disease with elevated left atrial pressures. Such varices resolve with mitral valve replacement.
▶ CTA demonstrates a vascular lesion in continuity with the pulmonary vein. Its enhancement matches that of the left atrium. PVVs are usually located within a few centimeters of the left atrium. The surrounding pulmonary arterial branches are normal.
▶ PVVs tend to stay stable in size, but they can grow if there is increased pulmonary venous hypertension due to worsening valvular disease.
▶ Complications are exceedingly rare and include thrombosis leading to systemic emboli, hemopericardium or hemothorax due to rupture into the pericardium or pleura, respectively, and rupture into a bronchus causing hemoptysis.
▶ Very rarely, a PVV can be confused with an inferior pulmonic pericardial recess on nonenhanced imaging.

Management

▶ As complications from PVV are exceedingly rare, treatment is usually not warranted.

Further Reading

Grassi FT, Bradshaw DA. A 28-year-old female with a right perihilar mass. *Respiration.* 2006;73:840-843.
Vanherreweghe E, Rigauts H, Bogaerts Y, et al. Pulmonary vein varix: diagnosis with multi-slice helical CT. *Eur Radiol.* 2000;10:1315-1317.

History

▸ 55-year-old man who underwent right knee amputation after a motor vehicle collision 2 days prior.

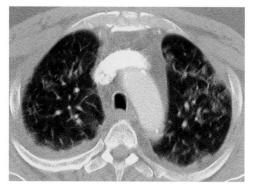

Figure 124.1

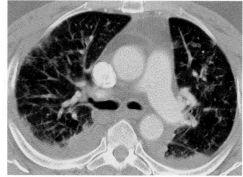

Figure 124.2

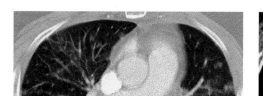

Figure 124.3

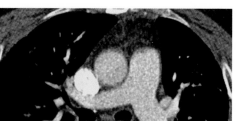

Figure 124.4

Case 124 Fat Emboli

Figure 124.5

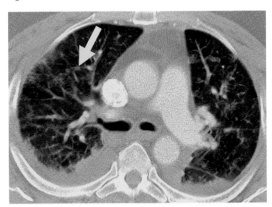

Findings

▶ CT shows multiple small ill-defined ground-glass nodular opacities, mostly located in the periphery of the lungs and closely associated with arteriolar endings (Figs. 124.1–124.3; arrow in Fig. 124.5).

▶ No pulmonary embolism is detected in the soft-tissue window setting (Fig. 124.4). There are small bilateral pleural effusions.

Differential Diagnosis

▶ The differential diagnosis for small ground-glass nodules associated with the centrilobular structures is usually led by tree-in-bud (TIB) from small airways diseases. In this case, the TIB-like finding is due to a vascular cause. Vascular TIB-like change can be from microemboli (fat, amniotic, tumor), pulmonary hypertension, or vasculitis. The history of long bone trauma allows for the fat embolism to move to the top of the list.

Teaching Points

▶ Fat embolism is usually seen in those who have sustained long bone fractures or have had intramedullary orthopedic procedures. It usually has a delayed onset of 12 to 72 hours.

▶ Fat embolism syndrome refers to a triad of acute respiratory failure and hypoxemia, neurologic deterioration, and petechiae.

▶ Deposition of fat within pulmonary capillaries leads to liberation of free fatty acids as the fat molecules break down. The fatty acids invoke an inflammatory response—a terminal pneumonitis.

▶ The fatty acids are not filtered by the lung because of their small size and lead to systemic embolization.

▶ Chest radiographic and CT imaging findings are nonspecific and may be similar to any cause of noncardiogenic pulmonary edema.

▶ A suggestive CT finding is the presence of multiple sub-centimeter ground-glass nodules. The ground-glass nodules tend to be subpleural and centrilobular and frequently demonstrate upper lung predominance.

▶ On CTA there are no filling defects in the pulmonary arteries and no fat density in the pulmonary infiltrates.

Management

▶ Management is mainly supportive. Measures are made to improve pulmonary function. If symptoms are severe, patients are mechanically ventilated. Most cases are self-limited. Rarely, patients will develop diffuse alveolar damage and adult respiratory distress syndrome (ARDS).

Further Reading

Gallardo X, Castaner E, Mata JM, et al. Nodular pattern at lung computed tomography in fat embolism syndrome: a helpful finding. *J Comput Assist Tomogr.* 2006;30:254-257.

History

▶ 57-year-old man with no known past medical disease complains of left-sided chest pain (worse on inspiration). He was found to be hypoxemic.

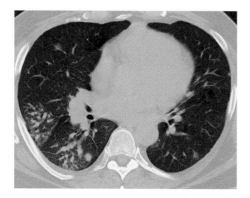

Figure 125.1

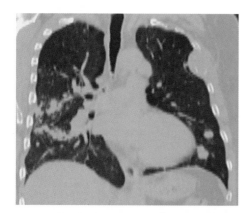

Figure 125.2

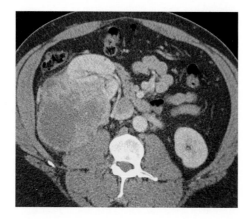

Figure 125.3

Case 125 Pulmonary Arterial Tumor Emboli

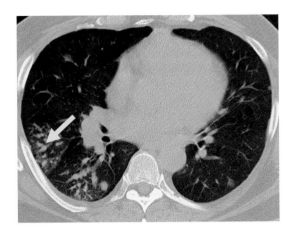

Figure 125.4

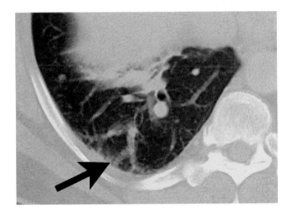

Figure 125.5

Findings

- CT demonstrates a beaded appearance of the distal arterial branches in the right lower and middle lobes, creating a mimic of tree-in-bud (TIB)(arrow in Fig. 125.4).
- Coronal reformation shows the nodularity of the bronchovascular bundles, in addition to well-circumscribed pulmonary nodules in the lingula and right lower lobe, and a lytic lesion involving the left fourth rib.
- Image of the upper abdomen (Fig. 125.3) shows a large mass arising from the left kidney, consistent with renal cell carcinoma.

Differential Diagnosis

- TIB nodules and associated branching densities are most commonly caused by bronchiolar or airway disease. Vascular mimics of TIB may be from microemboli (tumor, amniotic, or fat) or vasculitis. Recognizing the renal mass should help to make this rare diagnosis.

Teaching Points

- *Pulmonary arterial tumor emboli* refers to an occlusion of the arterioles by microemboli. Occasionally, large pulmonary artery filling defects may simultaneously be seen from macroscopic tumor emboli.

- On CT the distention of the small arterial branches creates the appearance of enlarged sausage-like peripheral arterioles (Fig. 125.5). The beaded look of the arteriole becomes more obvious as the disease advances, creating a mimic of TIB.
- Pulmonary tumor thrombotic microangiopathy is a rare form of tumor embolism where fibrocellular intimal hyperplasia of the arteries develops in response to embolized tumor cells, inciting thrombosis. On CT it appears as ground-glass centrilobular nodules.
- Concomitant septal line thickening due to lymphangitic carcinomatosis and peripheral wedge-shaped ground-glass opacities are common CT findings.
- Adenocarcinomas (breast, renal, adrenal, hepatocellular, gastric, colon) are the most common cancers leading to tumor emboli.
- Affected individuals present with progressive dyspnea and are found to have signs of pulmonary hypertension and severe hypoxemia.
- Tumor emboli is usually a sign of advanced metastasis and portends a grave prognosis.

Management

- There is no specific treatment for pulmonary artery tumor emboli.

Further Reading

Bhalla S, Lopez-Costa I. MDCT of acute thrombotic and nonthrombotic pulmonary emboli. *Eur J Radiol.* 2007;64:54-64.
Jorens PG, Van Marck E, Snoeckx A, et al. Nonthrombotic pulmonary embolism. *Eur Respir J.* 2009;34:452-457.

History

▶ 35-year-old man presents with progressive shortness of breath over the past 18 months.

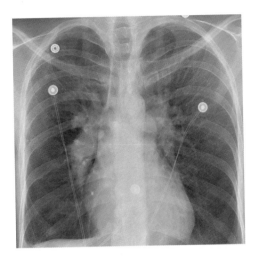

Figure 126.1

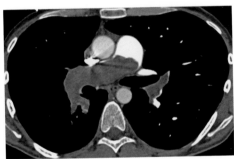

Figure 126.2

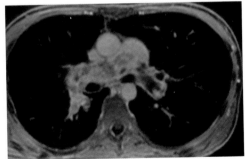

Figure 126.3

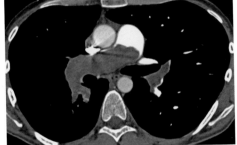

Figure 126.4

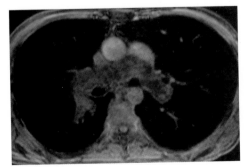

Figure 126.5

Case 126 Pulmonary Artery Sarcoma

Figure 126.6

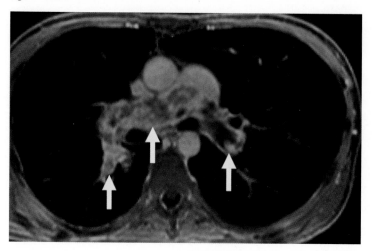

Findings

▶ Chest radiograph (Fig. 126.1) shows marked enlargement of the pulmonary arteries and their branches, especially the right interlobar artery.

▶ CTA (Figs. 126.2 and 126.3) reveals near-complete filling of the main and bilateral pulmonary arteries by a mostly low-attenuation lesion. The artery is expanded by this lesion (Fig. 126.2).

▶ This lesion shows progressive enhancement after gadolinium administration on thoracic MRA (arrows in Fig. 126.6).

Differential Diagnosis

▶ The differential diagnosis for a large intraluminal filling defect of the pulmonary arteries includes acute pulmonary embolism, tumor embolism, primary pulmonary artery neoplasm, and in situ thrombus. Given the long history of symptoms, lack of congenital heart disease, young age, and lesion enhancement, a primary artery neoplasm would be favored.

Teaching Points

▶ Pulmonary artery (PA) sarcoma is a rare malignant tumor arising from the intimal layer and is the most common primary tumor of the PAs.

▶ Most arise from the dorsal aspect of the main PA, and they tend to grow in the direction of blood flow.

▶ PA sarcoma occurs mostly in adults, with a mean age of diagnosis of 48 years.

▶ Clinical symptoms are nonspecific and variable.

▶ CTA demonstrates a low-attenuation mass that expands the artery and extends into many branches. The lesion may have regions of enhancement. Secondary findings include enlarged bronchial arteries, right ventricular hypertrophy, right atrial enlargement, and a patent foramen ovale.

▶ Enhancement of the lesion may be better visualized on gadolinium-enhanced MRA (Fig. 126.6).

▶ The asymmetric perfusion of the pulmonary arteries leads to mismatched ventilation-perfusion on scintigraphy, usually involving an entire lobe or lung.

- ▶ Definitive diagnosis is by biopsy. Since thrombi commonly accompany the sarcoma, sampling from various areas should be performed.
- ▶ The prognosis is very poor, with a mean survival rate of 12 to 18 months.

Management

- ▶ Surgical removal, usually by endarterectomy, is performed as a means to prolong life. The role of chemotherapy and radiation therapy is not clearly defined.

Further Reading

Viana-Tejedor A, Mariño-Enríquez A, Sánchez-Recalde A, et al. Intimal sarcoma of the pulmonary artery: diagnostic value of different imaging techniques. *Rev Esp Cardiol.* 2008;61(12):1355-1365.

Part 14 Thoracic Trauma and Emergent Aortic Conditions

History

▶ 32-year-old man with hypertension is admitted to the Emergency Department.

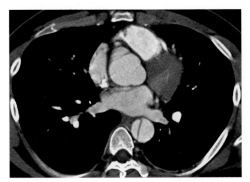

Figure 127.1

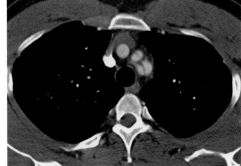

Figure 127.2

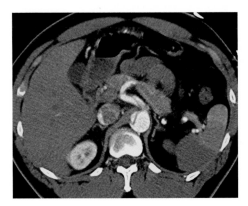

Figure 127.3

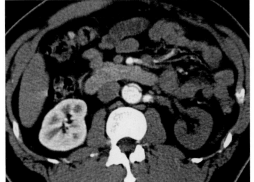

Figure 127.4

Case 127 Aortic Dissection (Stanford Type A)

Figure 127.5

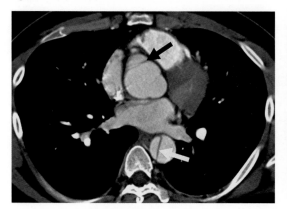

Figure 127.6

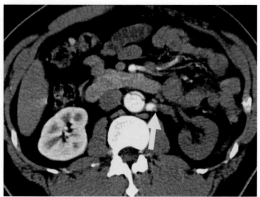

Findings

▶ CTA shows linear hypodensities in the aorta (arrows in Fig. 127.5) consistent with a dissection intimomedial flap.
▶ The dissection extends into the left common carotid, left subclavian (Fig. 127.2), and celiac arteries, with no enhancement of the posterior half of the spleen. (Fig. 127.3).
▶ The left renal artery has an abrupt cutoff (arrow in Fig. 127.6) with resultant absent renal enhancement.

Differential Diagnosis

▶ The flap in the descending aorta identifies an aortic dissection (AD) but the ascending aortic finding could be a flap or pulsation artifact on a non-gated study. The clarity of the finding and the lack of artifact within the right ventricle outflow make pulsation unlikely.

Teaching Points

▶ AD results from a tear in the aortic intima, creating a false passage within the media.
▶ Predisposing conditions for AD include hypertension (most common cause in elderly patients), Marfan syndrome (most common cause in patients <40 years old), bicuspid aortopathy, pregnancy, cocaine use, and iatrogenic trauma to the aorta.
▶ The Stanford classification is based on the location of aortic involvement. Type A dissection involves the aorta proximal to the origin of the left subclavian artery (LSCA). Type B dissections begin distal to the LSCA.
▶ Type A dissections are at higher risk of aortic rupture and can extend into the aortic root, coronary arteries, and pericardium.
▶ Type B dissections propagate distally and can obstruct vessels to the abdominal organs and lower extremities, leading to ischemia.
▶ Chest radiography is quite nonspecific and should not be used to exclude AD.
▶ CTA will readily demonstrate the intimal flap.
▶ The false lumen tends to be larger than the true lumen. It may contain strands of media (cobweb sign) and create an acute angle between the flap and wall (beak sign) (arrow in Fig. 127.6).

Management

▶ Type A dissections are repaired immediately.
▶ Type B dissections are initially managed medically with blood pressure control.
▶ Type B aortic dissections that rupture, occlude a major branch artery, or grow require emergent surgery.

Further Reading

Yoo SM, Lee HY, White CS. MDCT evaluation of acute aortic syndromes. *Radiol Clin North Am.* 2010 Jan;48(1):67-83.

History

▶ 72-year-old woman with hypertension is admitted with chest pain.

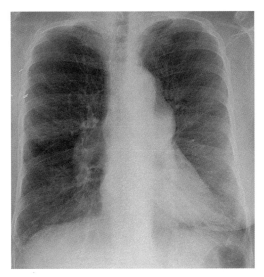

Figure 128.1

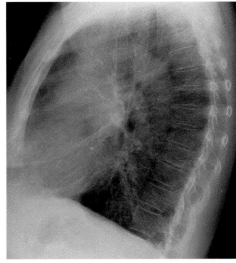

Figure 128.2

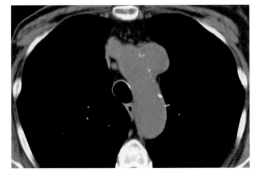

Figure 128.3

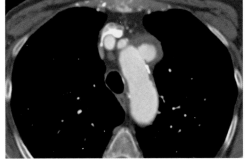

Figure 128.4

Case 128 Penetrating Atherosclerotic Ulcer (PAU)

Findings

- Chest radiograph shows an abnormal convexity between the aorta and pulmonary artery, most notable on the frontal view (Fig. 128.1).
- Unenhanced CT shows a focal, lateral outpouching of the aortic arch separated from the aortic lumen by intimal calcifications (Fig. 128.2).
- Contrast confirms that the outpouching communicates with the lumen and has crater-like edges. The saccular outpouching is associated with aortic atherosclerosis and a peripheral hematoma.

Differential Diagnosis

- The differential diagnosis for saccular outpouching of the aorta in this location includes a penetrating atherosclerotic ulcer (PAU) or a mycotic aortic aneurysm. The outpouching is slightly proximal to the usual location of post-traumatic pseudoaneurysms or ductus aneurysms.

Teaching Points

- PAU develops when an atheromatous plaque ulcerates beyond the intima, allowing the lumen to communicate with the media.
- The PAU may regress, rupture, or progress by leading to an intramural hematoma (IMH), dissection, or a focal, saccular pseudoaneurysm.
- The risk of aortic rupture is higher with PAU than with a classical dissection.
- Care must be taken to avoid confusing an ulcerated atherosclerotic plaque with a PAU. When acute, PAUs present with chest pain.
- PAUs are mostly located in the middle and distal third of the descending thoracic aorta; PAU of the ascending aorta is rare.
- Typically patients with PAUs are hypertensive, elderly patients with atherosclerosis of the aorta.
- On CT and MR, a PAU appears as a contrast-filled crater-like focal outpouching that communicates with the lumen. A variable amount of IMH is seen.

Management

- Most PAUs are managed medically as their presence is indicative of a diseased, fragile aorta.
- Pain, hemodynamic instability, rapid expansion of aortic diameter, increasing aortic wall thickness, and a size larger than 20 mm in diameter and 10 mm in depth are all indicators for surgical repair, most commonly by endovascular stent grafting.

Further Reading

Castañer E, Andreu M, Gallardo X, et al. CT in nontraumatic acute thoracic aortic disease: typical and atypical features and complications. *Radiographics*. 2003 Oct;23 Spec No:S93-110.

Hayashi H, Matsuoka Y, Sakamoto I, et al. Penetrating atherosclerotic ulcer of the aorta: imaging features and disease concept. *Radiographics*. 2000 Jul-Aug;20(4):995-1005.

History

▶ 67-year-old woman with aortic aneurysm presents with sharp central chest pain.

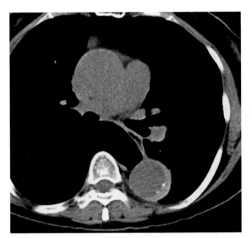

Figure 129.1

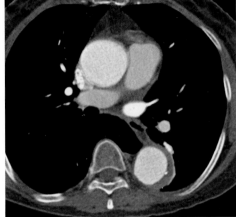

Figure 129.2

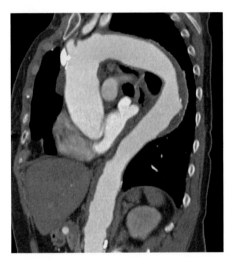

Figure 129.3

Case 129   Acute Intramural Hematoma (IMH)

Figure 129.4

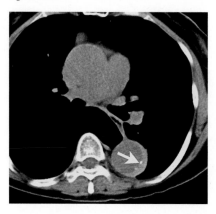

Findings

▶ Unenhanced (Fig. 129.1) and contrast-enhanced (Fig. 129.2) CT images show a hyperattenuating and nonenhancing crescent-shaped thickening of the descending aortic wall. This thickening displaces the intimal calcification toward the lumen (arrow in Fig. 129.4).

▶ CT reconstruction shows the craniocaudal extent of this lesion, which results in fusiform dilatation of the affected portion of the aorta (Fig. 129.3).

Differential Diagnosis

▶ The differential diagnosis for crescentic aortic thickening includes an aortic intramural hematoma (IMH), atherosclerosis, and a thrombosed false lumen in an aortic dissection. The high attenuation on the noncontrast image would favor IMH. Aortitis can result in aortic thickening but is usually circumferential.

Teaching Points

▶ IMH refers to blood within the aortic media.

▶ Primary IMH is from spontaneous hemorrhage of the vaso vasorum without rupture of the intima.

▶ A penetrating atherosclerotic ulcer can also result in an IMH.

▶ Systemic hypertension is the leading risk factor for the development of an IMH.

▶ IMH is responsible for 13% to 20% of all acute aortic syndromes.

▶ Unenhanced CT shows eccentric thickening of the aortic wall, displacing the intimal calcifications medially. When the IMH is acute, the attenuation of the thickening is higher than blood pool but not as high as calcium.

▶ An IMH should not enhance with intravenous contrast.

▶ T2-weighted MR shows high signal of the thrombus in acute IMH, which decreases with time.

▶ Occasionally, areas of contrast blush may be seen in an IMH. These have been attributed to flow from intercostal or bronchial arteries and are associated with decreased likelihood of spontaneous IMH regression.

▶ IMH may regress, rupture, or develop a communication with the lumen and establish flow in the media (dissection).

Management

▶ If the IMH involves the ascending aorta, it is usually managed surgically.

▶ Descending aorta involvement alone can be managed conservatively with control of hypertension. Since progression of the IMH occurs mostly in the first month after presentation, close monitoring with serial transesophageal echocardiography, CT, or MR is performed.

Further Reading

Chao CP, Walker TG, Kalva SP. Natural history and CT appearances of aortic intramural hematoma. *Radiographics*. 2009 May-Jun; 29(3):791-804.

History

► 29-year-old woman is admitted after a high-speed motor vehicle collision.

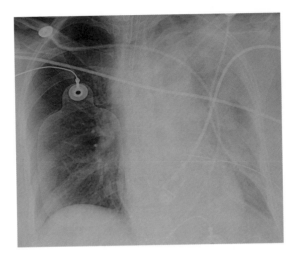

Figure 130.1

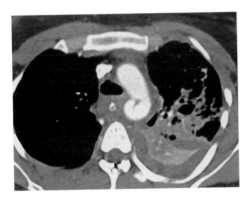

Figure 130.2

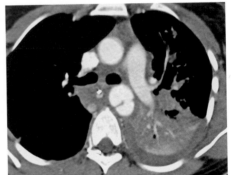

Figure 130.3

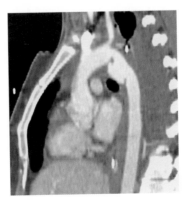

Figure 130.4

Case 130 Acute Traumatic Aortic Injury (TAI)

Figure 130.5

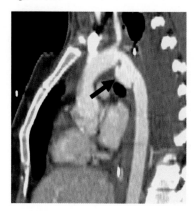

Findings

▸ Chest radiograph (Fig. 130.1) shows a wide mediastinum, displacement of the endotracheal and nagogastric tubes to the right, and an indistinct aortic contour.

▸ CTA (Figs. 130.2–130.4) confirms the presence of a mediastinal hematoma and reveals a saccular outpouching of the aortic isthmus (arrow in Fig. 130.5). Left hemothorax and pulmonary contusions are also seen.

Differential Diagnosis

▸ The differential diagnosis for saccular outpouching of the aortic isthmus consists of a post-traumatic aortic injury (TAI) or a ductus aneurysm. The mediastinal blood and the history of trauma make the former diagnosis the only plausible one.

Teaching Points

▸ TAI occurs from differential deceleration in the setting of blunt trauma. This differential shearing causes the aortic wall to rupture, commonly at sites where the aorta is tacked to adjacent structures, such as the aortic root, the aortic isthmus, the diaphragmatic hiatus, and the origins of the three main vascular branches.

▸ Of those who survive their trauma, the aortic isthmus is the most common site of TAI.

▸ Radiographic findings of TAI include mediastinal widening, indistinct aortic contour, rightward deviation of the trachea and nasogastric tube, inferior displacement of the left mainstem bronchus, and left apical capping.

▸ CT findings of TAI can be divided into direct and indirect signs. An indirect sign refers to mediastinal blood that effaces the fat plane with the aorta and warrants further investigation.

▸ Direct signs include a linear filling defect, eccentric thrombus, abnormal aortic contour, abrupt change in aortic contour, or active extravasation. These findings prompt immediate treatment and do not require confirmatory testing. *Patients with direct signs of TAI should go directly to treatment.*

▸ Approximately 2% of untreated TAI cases present as a chronic pseudoaneurysm. These are frequently treated to prevent latent rupture.

Management

▸ Most cases of TAI will be immediately repaired. Increasingly, endovascular techniques are used.

▸ Rarely, CT will demonstrate a minimal aortic injury (MAI) such as eccentric thrombus without any other finding. This MAI may be treated with beta-blocker therapy alone or may be treated after the non-aortic injuries are addressed.

Further Reading

Creasy JD, Chiles C, Routh WD, et al. Overview of traumatic injury of the thoracic aorta. *Radiographics*. 1997 Jan-Feb;17(1):27-45.

History

▶ 76-year-old woman underwent laparoscopic cholecystectomy. Immediately after extubation, she complained of chest pain and face swelling.

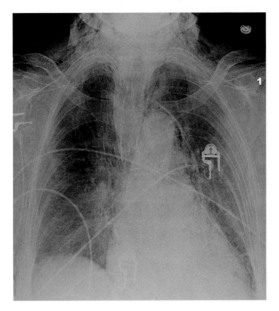

Figure 131.1

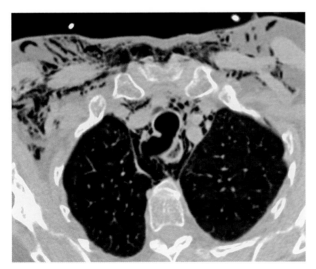

Figure 131.2

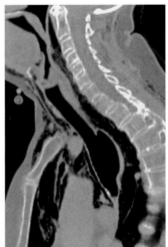

Figure 131.3

Case 131 Tracheobronchial Injury

Figure 131.4

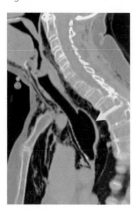

Figure 131.5

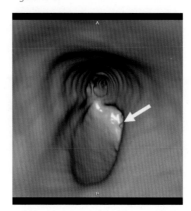

Findings

▶ Chest radiograph demonstrates pneumomediastinum and extensive subcutaneous emphysema.

▶ CT demonstrates an extraluminal air collection immediately posterior to the trachea, closely associated with a defect along the posterior tracheal wall, which can be seen on endoluminal volume-rendered image (arrow in Figs. 131.4 and 131.5).

Differential Diagnosis

▶ A tracheal diverticulum (from cartilaginous defect or due to chronic obstructive lung disease) is the main alternative. A diverticulum can perforate upon coughing. In this case, the history makes a tracheal injury most likely.

Teaching Points

▶ Acute tracheobronchial injury (TBI) is rare, occurring in about 1.5% of major blunt trauma cases. It can also occur after intubation.

▶ TBI is caused by partial or complete tear of the airway wall.

▶ About one third of patients die within the first 2 hours after trauma.

▶ Clinical diagnosis is delayed in 50% of patients due to a low clinical suspicion. The most common symptoms are dyspnea and hemoptysis.

▶ Delayed clinical presentation usually occurs mostly after 4 weeks, with symptoms of hemoptysis or mediastinitis. The ensuing fibrosis with healing leads to airway stenosis. This can cause recurrent pneumonia, chronic atelectasis, and lung collapse.

▶ In blunt trauma most TBI injuries occur within 2.5 cm of the carina. The defect is usually at the junction of the cartilaginous and membranous portions of the airway wall.

▶ Imaging findings of TBI include extensive pneumomediastinum leading to subcutaneous emphysema, progressive pneumothorax that does not resolve after placement of a correctly positioned chest tube, and lung collapse towards the diaphragm (upright) or posterolateral chest wall (supine), creating the *fallen lung sign*.

▶ Posterior or lateral herniation of the endotracheal tube or its balloon, defect in the tracheobronchial wall, and irregularity of the tracheobronchial wall are CT findings of TBI.

▶ Multiplanar and volume-rendered images are helpful in guiding bronchoscopy and in surgical planning.

Management

▶ Confirmation of the airway injury by bronchoscopy is a common practice.

▶ The airway wall defect must be surgically repaired to prevent complications.

Further Reading

Scaglione M, Romanoa S, Pinto A, et al. Acute tracheobronchial injuries: impact of imaging on diagnosis and management implications. *Eur J Radiol.* 2006;59:336-343.

History

▶ 17-year-old male presents with right chest pain after an all-terrain-vehicle accident.

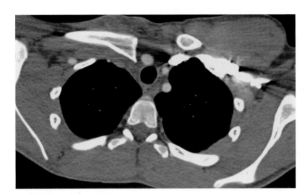

Figure 132.1

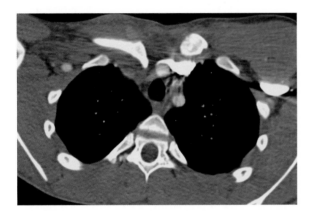

Figure 132.2

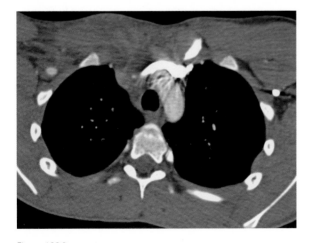

Figure 132.3

Case 132 Posterior Sternoclavicular Joint Dislocation

Figure 132.4

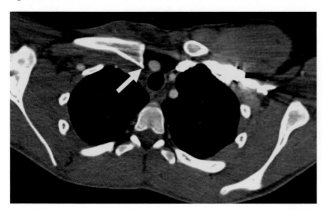

Figure 132.5

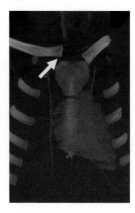

Findings

▶ The right clavicular head is displaced posteriorly (arrows in Figs. 132.4 and 132.5) into the mediastinum with associated soft tissue swelling and stranding. Note the close relationship of the displaced clavicular head to the brachiocephalic artery (which was not injured in this case).

Differential Diagnosis

▶ There should be no differential diagnosis.

Teaching Points

▶ Resulting from direct blunt trauma to the sternum or lateral blunt trauma to the ipsilateral shoulder, the direction of dislocation is thought to be related to the position of the acromion compared to the manubrium at the time of impact. Anterior dislocation is more common as the acromion is usually posterior to the manubrium at the time of injury and the posterior joint capsule is better formed than the anterior portion.

▶ Both types can present with pain and swelling at the joint site as well as limited mobility of the shoulder.

▶ Approximately 25% to 30% of posterior sternoclavicular dislocations are associated with complications, which result from displacement of the medial clavicle into the mediastinum. Vascular injuries, such as laceration or dissection, can occur to the subclavian artery or vein, brachiocephalic artery or vein, common carotid artery, and superior vena cava. Tracheal compression can also occur as well as upper extremity nerve damage.

▶ Diagnosis depends on CT imaging. CT allows for assessment of the dislocation and any potential complications. If possible, intravenous contrast should be administered via the opposite upper extremity to prevent streak artifact from dense contrast inflow from obscuring vascular assessment.

Management

▶ In both anterior and posterior sternoclavicular dislocations, closed reduction is the first line of treatment. If unsuccessful, especially in cases of posterior dislocation, open surgical relocation may be required.

Further Reading

Jaggard MK, Gupte CM, Gulati V, Reilly P. A comprehensive review of trauma and disruption to the sternoclavicular joint with the proposal of a new classification system. *J Trauma*. 2009 Feb;66(2):576-584.

Kaewlai R, Avery LL, Asrani AV, Novelline RA. Multidetector CT of blunt thoracic trauma. *Radiographics*. 2008 Oct;28(6):1555-1570.

History

► 55-year-old man with hemoptysis and a history of coronary artery bypass surgery is admitted for chest pain.

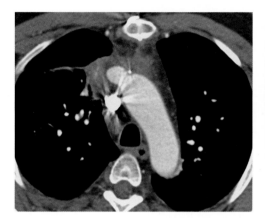

Figure 133.1

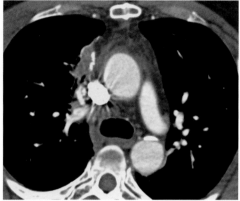

Figure 133.2

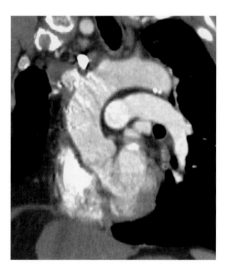

Figure 133.3

Case 133 Aortotomy Pseudoaneurysm (PSA)

Figure 133.4

Figure 133.5

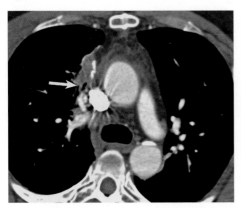
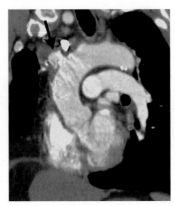

Findings

▶ CT images (Figs. 133.1 and 133.3) show a contrast-filled focal outpouching arising from the anterior wall of the ascending aorta. It is surrounded by high-attenuation material consistent with a hematoma (arrows in Figs. 133.4 and 133.5). Note that the outpouching is closer to the great vessels than the aortic root.

Differential Diagnosis

▶ A focal outpouching of the ascending aorta in a patient who has undergone coronary bypass may be from an aortotomy (prior aortic cannulation site) pseudoaneurysm (PSA) or from a complication of the bypass graft (thrombosed graft or anastomotic PSA). The location (2 cm caudal to the innominate artery) would favor an aortotomy PSA.

Teaching Points

▶ PSAs of the ascending aorta occur when one or more layers of the aortic wall are disrupted, and the outpouching is contained by fewer than three layers of the aortic wall.

▶ After median sternotomy, a PSA may develop at an aortotomy site, a bypass graft anastomosis, or an aortic anastomosis in patients who have undergone ascending aortic repair or aortic valve repair. Location within the ascending aorta can be key in distinguishing among the types of PSAs.

▶ Infection is a predisposing factor for the development of a PSA.

▶ Small PSAs cause no symptoms. When large, they compress adjacent structures and may result in a hemopericardium.

▶ Diagnosis is made by CTA, which demonstrates the PSA surrounded by a hematoma of variable size.

▶ Post-processing with thin maximum intensity projections, volume-rendering, and multiplanar reformations can be helpful in identifying the site of origin.

Management

▶ A medium to large aortotomy PSA is considered a surgical urgency or emergency.

▶ In the era of routine cross-sectional imaging, small PSAs are often incidentally detected. These may be followed if they are asymptomatic and no signs of hemorrhage are observed.

Further Reading

Gabbieri D, Dohmen PM, Linneweber J, et al. Mycotic pseudoaneurysm of the ascending aorta at site of aortic cannulation. *Asian Cardiovasc Thorac Ann.* 2008 Apr;16(2):e15-17.

Nakayama T, Saito T, Asano M, et al. An aneurysm at the cannulation site discovered 40 years after cardiac surgery: report of a case. *Ann Thorac Cardiovasc Surg.* 2008 Aug;14(4):267-269.

Part 15   Postsurgical Cases

History

► 10-year-old boy who underwent bilateral lung transplant 3 years earlier presents with increasing shortness of breath and cough over the past month.

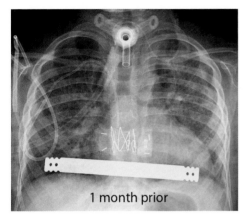

Figure 134.1

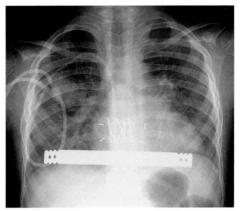

Figure 134.2

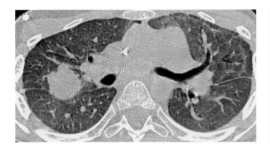

Figure 134.3

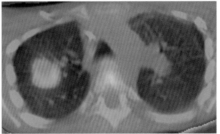

Figure 134.4

Case 134 Post-transplant Lymphoproliferative Disorder (PTLD)

Findings

- Surgical changes from lung transplantation and pectus repair are noted on the chest radiographs.
- Interval development of a mass lesion in the right upper lobe over 1 month can also be seen in the series of radiographs.
- The mass is well circumscribed on CT (Fig. 134.3) with some air bronchograms and shows moderate FDG uptake on PET (Fig. 134.4)

Differential Diagnosis

- Infection (bacterial vs. fungal) or post-transplant lymphoproliferative disease (PTLD) would head the differential diagnosis in this post-lung transplant patient.

Teaching Points

- PTLD can develop very rapidly, unlike most pulmonary neoplastic processes.
- PTLD represents a heterogeneous group of diseases, ranging from polyclonal lymphoid hyperplasia to monoclonal malignant lymphoma. Risk factors affecting the incidence of PTLD include presence of Epstein-Barr infection, allograft type, and degree of immunosuppression.
- PTLD comes from unregulated lymphoid expansion related to the chronic immunosuppression and is seen more commonly in multi-organ transplant recipients and in patients with more intensive immunosuppression, such as heart and/or lung transplant patients.
- Frequency of thoracic involvement varies with allograft type: in lung transplant patients, thoracic involvement is present in >60% of cases.
- Parenchymal involvement is four times more common than mediastinal node involvement.
- Appearance in the lung varies from discrete nodules to airspace consolidation.
- PTLD usually manifests as solitary or multiple nodules about 1 to 4 cm in size. They are usually well circumscribed, but may have a halo, and are usually solid but may cavitate.
- Airspace consolidation may be a manifestation of PTLD and is frequently multifocal akin to infection.

Management

- Most patients are asymptomatic in the early stages of the disease. Clinical symptoms will guide the clinician, since currently there is no role for imaging in screening asymptomatic patients.
- The initial treatment is reduction of immunosuppression, which is especially effective in early polyclonal lesions. Chemotherapy is the mainstay of treatment in monoclonal lesions and in lesions that are unresponsive to immunosuppression reduction.

Further Reading

Borhani AA, Hosseinzadeh K, Almusa O, et al. Imaging of posttransplantation lymphoproliferative disorder after solid organ transplantation. *Radiographics.* 2009;29:981-1002.

History

▶ 62-year-old woman presents with wheezing and dyspnea 1 year after a right pneumonectomy.

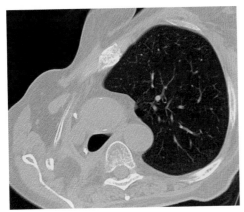

Figure 135.1

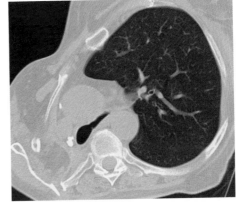

Figure 135.2

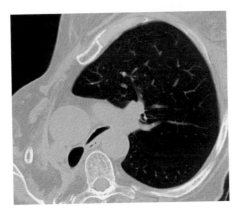

Figure 135.3

Case 135   Post-pneumonectomy Syndrome

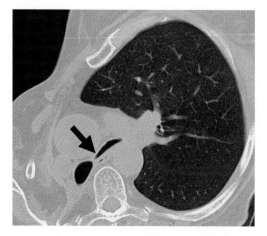

Figure 135.4

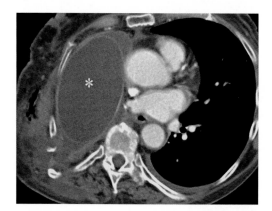

Figure 135.5

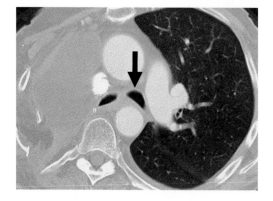

Figure 135.6

Findings

▶ Initial CT shows the marked right volume loss, in keeping with the patient's history of pneumonectomy. Note the accompanying narrowing of the left mainstem bronchus (arrow in Fig. 135.4).

▶ Subsequent CT, performed 1 month later, shows a breast implant used to reposition the mediastinum (asterisk in Fig. 135.5). The left mainstem bronchus (arrow in Fig. 135.6) is no longer narrowed.

Differential Diagnosis

▶ Differential diagnosis based on time course after surgery would include recurrent tumor, tracheal or esophageal fistulae to the pleura, indolent infection, or post-pneumonectomy syndrome. Once the CT is performed, no differential should exist.

Teaching Points

▶ Post-pneumonectomy syndrome is a delayed complication seen about 1 year after pneumonectomy, usually on the opposite side of the aortic arch. The volume loss results in stretching of the mainstem bronchus and compression of the trachea between the remaining pulmonary artery and the aorta.

▶ Patients usually have exertional dyspnea, inspiratory stridor, and recurrent pulmonary infections.

▶ Frequently, tracheobronchomalacia also develops, compounding the clinical symptoms.

▶ CT is the best method to diagnose post-pneumonectomy syndrome and will show abnormal narrowing of the distal part of the trachea and the mainstem bronchus between the pulmonary artery anteriorly and the aorta and spine posteriorly.

Management

▶ Various surgical procedures have been used to reposition the mediastinum. Silicone breast implants have been used in the post-pneumonectomy space to reposition the mediastinum. In adults, the results have been variable. In this case, the patient had to be stented as well.

Further Reading

Chae EJ, Seo JB, Kim SY, et al. Radiographic and CT findings of thoracic complications after pneumonectomy. *Radiographics*. 2006 Sep-Oct;26(5):1449-1468.

History

▶ Intensive care unit radiograph is obtained 2 weeks after an aortic repair.

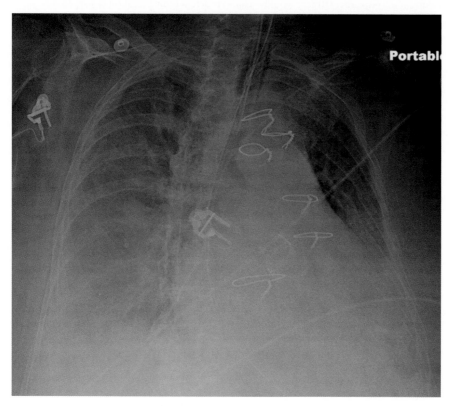

Figure 136.1

Case 136   Sternal Dehiscence

Figure 136.2

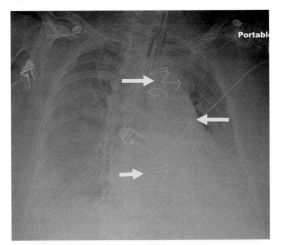

Figure 136.3

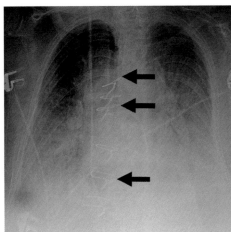

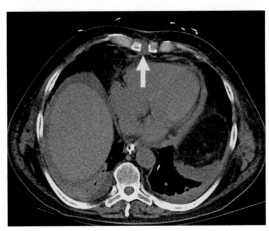

Figure 136.4

Findings

- Portable chest radiograph shows offset of the sternal wires (arrows in Fig. 136.2), which do not form a straight vertical line. This is more obvious when compared to the immediate postoperative study (Fig. 136.3).
- The migration of the sternal wires can easily be overlooked in the setting of the other catheters and the mild pulmonary edema.
- CT performed shortly after confirms the sternal dehiscence (arrow in Fig. 136.4).

Differential Diagnosis

- The malposition of the sternal wires should have no differential diagnosis. Though rotation can move the wires to one side of the sternum, they should retain their vertical linear relationship.

Teaching Points

- Sternal wires should not migrate after surgery. When they do, the question of dehiscence must be raised.
- Radiographic features of dehiscence usually precede clinical suspicion by 3 days on average.

- Radiographic findings are often the initial indication that sternal dehiscence is developing. By the time sternal breakdown is clinically evident, infection, abscess, and osteomyelitis may be well advanced.
- There is an approximate 20% mortality rate for sternal dehiscence, which is seen in about 1% to 2% of patients undergoing median sternotomy.
- The risk of dehiscence increases in obese patients, diabetics, and individuals with grafts involving both the left internal mammary and the right internal mammary arteries.

Management

- As dehiscence is almost always not clinically evident, a call to the clinician is necessary to alert them to sternal breakdown.
- CT is usually performed to evaluate for abscess, osteomyelitis, and mediastinitis.
- Treatment is based on the severity of findings and can include antibiotics, débridement, or sternectomy.

Further Reading

Boiselle PM, Mansilla AV, Fisher MS, McLoud TC. Wandering wires: frequency of sternal wire abnormalities in patients with sternal dehiscence. *AJR Am J Roentgenol.* 1999 Sep;173(3):777-780.

History

▸ 64-year-old man immediately after an esophagectomy receives this chest radiograph.

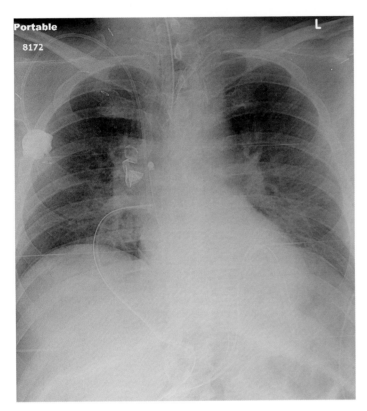

Figure 137.1

Case 137   Retained Laparotomy Sponge

Figure 137.2

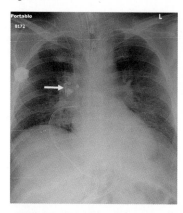

Figure 137.3

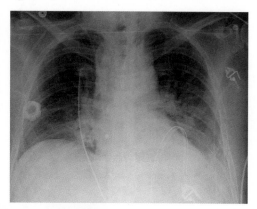

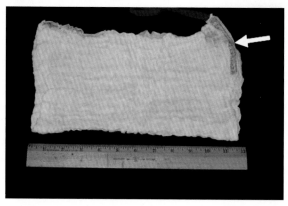

Figure 137.4

Findings

- Initial chest radiograph is in keeping with the intraoperative nature of this study. Endotracheal tube, Penrose drain at the thoracic inlet, port catheter, chest tubes, and mediastinal drain are all in expected positions. An unexpected ribbon-like opacity is seen in the right hilar region (arrow in Fig. 137.2). This opacity is in keeping with a laparotomy sponge.
- The sponge is no longer seen on the follow-up radiograph (Fig. 137.3).
- Photograph of another similar sponge shows the blue, radiopaque marker (arrow in Fig. 137.4).

Differential Diagnosis

- There should be no differential diagnosis.

Teaching Points

- A retained surgical sponge is often referred to as a *gossypiboma* (*gossypium* [Latin, cotton] and *boma* [Swahili, place of concealment]). However, as some packing may not be cotton, some prefer the more generic term *textiloma*.
- The likelihood of a retained sponge is higher in patients who have emergency surgery, an unexpected change in surgical procedure, or a higher mean body-mass index.
- In reported cases with retained sponges, sponge counts have been falsely correct in up to 76% of surgeries.

- In June 2005, the Joint Commission on Accreditation of Healthcare Organizations (JCAHO) added "unintended retention of a foreign object in an individual after surgery or other procedure" to the list of sentinel events that require hospitals to perform a root cause analysis and report the event to the JCAHO registry.
- As of October 2008, Medicare started denying payment for 10 "reasonably preventable" conditions, including second operations to retrieve a retained sponge.
- Because of the potential to affect the accreditation and reimbursement for hospitals, many hospitals have started requiring the routine use of operative radiography to detect any retained sponge or surgical instrument.
- Undoubtedly, operative radiography will become a greater part of many hospital-based practices. As a result, it behooves all Radiologists to be familiar with the surgical sponges in use at their institutions.

Management
- When a retained sponge, gauze, or instrument is encountered on a radiograph, the Radiologist should immediately call the referring physician and document the discussion.
- These retained foreign bodies should be removed.

Further Reading
Cima RR, Kollengode A, Garnatz J, et al. Incidence and characteristics of potential and actual retained foreign object events in surgical patients. *J Am Coll Surg.* 2008 Jul;207(1):80-87.
Madan R, Trotman-Dickenson B, Hunsaker AR. Intrathoracic gossypiboma. *AJR Am J Roentgenol.* 2007 Aug;189(2):W90-91.
Wolfson KA, Seeger LL, Kadell BM, Eckardt JJ. Imaging of surgical paraphernalia: what belongs in the patient and what does not. *Radiographics.* 2000 Nov-Dec;20(6):1665-1673.

Index of Cases

Index